THE PFIZER GUIDE

NURSING CAREER OPPORTUNITIES

Edited by
Mary O. Mundinger, DrPH, RN
Dean
Columbia University School of Nursing
New York, New York

Editorial Board

The Pfizer Guide: Nursing Career Opportunities is published for the Pfizer Laboratories, Pratt, and Roerig divisions of Pfizer Inc, New York, NY, by Merritt Communications, Inc., copyright © 1994. The contents are determined independently and do not necessarily reflect the views of Pfizer Inc or the publisher. No part of this publication may be reproduced in any form without prior written permission from the publisher. Correspondence should be addressed to The Pfizer Guide, c/o Merritt Communications, Inc., 142 Ferry Road, Old Saybrook, CT 06475.

ISBN 1-885031-01-7

Printed in The United States of America

Pfizer Inc
235 East 42nd Street
New York, NY 10017-5755
Tel 212 573 2251 Fax 212 808 8652

Karen Katen
Vice President—Pfizer Inc
Executive Vice President—U.S. Pharmaceuticals Group

Dear Nursing Student:

Professional opportunities in nursing have multiplied rapidly during the past two decades and continue to increase each year.

To help the student nurse thread his or her own way through the maze of traditional and new directions in nursing, Pfizer has joined with leaders of the profession in launching this new guide to nursing careers. Here, successful nurses speak frankly of the challenges they have faced, the influences that have impacted their choice of specialty, and the prospects they see ahead.

We at Pfizer are pleased to sponsor this guide. We hope it will be a valuable aid for every nursing student in making critical decisions associated with career choice.

My best wishes for a long and successful professional career.

Sincerely,

Karen Katen

TABLE OF CONTENTS

INTRODUCTION

SPECIALTIES: AN OVERVIEW

Contents

Contents

OTHER PROFESSIONAL AREAS

Contents

MANAGEMENT

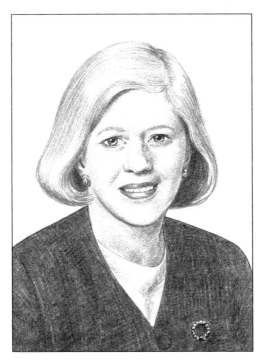

Mary O. Mundinger, DrPH, RN,
is dean of the Columbia University
School of Nursing,
New York, New York.

Nursing's Promising Future and Your Advanced Practice Choice

Only five generations of nurses have set their footprints in history since Florence Nightingale's pioneering work. In that short time, nursing has grown enormously in knowledge, skill, prestige, and value. Today, on the brink of a new millennium, scientists and policy makers recognize nursing as the health profession with the most untapped contributions for improving the health of our nation.

In this century, America witnessed nursing first as the courageous and visionary presence in home visiting and community-based care. Lifting their long skirts over tenement rooftops in New York City, hard-working public health nurses avoided the many flights up and down as they visited desperately poor young mothers and their newborns, terminally ill cancer and tuberculosis patients, and the frail elderly.

During World War I, nurses cared for patients on the European front and ran the hospitals at home, in the absence of their physician colleagues who were at war. The influenza epidemic was its own battlefield, where nurses and their care were often the critical ingredient in a patient's survival.

Recognizing that the social context was crucial to health, nurses opened soup kitchens during the Depression, counseled families about cheap but nutritious diets, and set up school health stations to tend to children otherwise neglected by the health care system. During the 1930s, American nurses continued to establish and provide most community-based care, except for physicians' house calls to the critically ill.

During World War II, nurses were among the first health professionals to arrive in Europe to staff field hospitals and nurture back to health injured, maimed, and emotionally scarred veterans. Nurses abandoned their uniforms for coveralls and GI shirts and pants, joining their medical colleagues in the indistinguishable teamwork of saving lives.

When these nurses sailed back to the United States, confident of their expertise and proud of their teamwork on the battlefield, they became part of a generation of American women who found that with the return of men to the work force, women were relegated to their prewar status. This happened in the civilian work force as well — Rosie the Riveter turned over her tools to the returning veteran and again took up her apron and labor in the kitchen.

The burgeoning hospital and the emergence of biomedical and technological breakthroughs marked the post-World War II era. Huge federal subsidies enabled hospitals to flourish, and all those new beds were a powerful magnet. More and more Americans were admitted to the hospital for illnesses that traditionally had been treated at home, and they were admitted for longer periods of time. In fact, it was not unusual for a patient with a minor heart attack to spend six to eight weeks in a hospital bed.

The insurance industry boomed during the 1950s, and in keeping with the belief that more is better, the amount of care given grew as did cost. Because most of its cost was tied to physician fees and hospital charges, the insurance industry helped entrench the belief that health care is medical care and that payment should go directly only to doctors and hospitals. During this same time, nursing essentially gained a monopoly on community-based care. Baccalaureate education in nursing began its ascendancy, with hospital-based, task-oriented diploma programs losing applicants. Baccalaureate education stressed public health nursing and leadership training, further advancing the BS nurse as the hospital team leader, or head nurse, or the one in the community who was the decision maker in home care.

The shortage of physicians during the war had virtually eliminated house calls; the remaining available physicians could see many more patients in a day if they came to the physicians' offices. The resulting increase in productivity also yielded higher financial rewards. In the void, nurses took up home visiting for patients who could not get to the doctor's office, but unlike other medical costs, home visiting was paid for through charitable organizations and individuals. Insurance companies that paid for physicians' house calls did not pay for nurses' house calls.

As a result, nurses became more and more concentrated in hospitals, where their salaried services were part of the aggregate per diem rate, along with dietary services, heat, and linen supplies. Admission to a hospital, except for the few hours that may be spent in surgery, places a patient almost entirely in the care of a nurse. Yet hospitals are not configured to protect and focus that nursing resource; increasingly hospitals are high-technology systems of care that have made the value of nursing largely invisible and, therefore, inadequately recognized and recompensed. A lesson was learned: That which is paid for directly is given the highest value. Nursing began to act on this axiom.

In the 1950s, nursing schools developed the first advanced practice programs in midwifery and psychiatric nursing at the graduate level. Other specialties proliferated in the 1960s, and in 1965 the promising and exciting new role of nurse practitioner (NP) was born.

Lee Ford, RN, and Henry Silver, MD, working together in professional collaboration in Colorado, recognized their community's unmet need for the health care of children. They developed an expanded public health nursing role, which involved diagnosing, treating, and managing uncomplicated health problems. The same year saw the passage of Medicare and Medicaid, two groundbreaking federal programs that insured payment for health care for the elderly and the poor. While nurse practitioners are specifically excluded from direct payment under the original statute, amendments during the ensuing 28 years have provided NPs greater access to federal payment for their services to these populations.

In the private sector, NPs gained direct reimbursement even faster as it soon became apparent that their services were of high quality, were predictable and broadly competent, and were cost effective. During these early years of NP development, the nation struggled under the Nixon administration's wage and price controls and, for the first time, the number of nurses working in hospitals was reduced and constrained. Nurses began to see that job security as well as fair remuneration would be tied to more independent roles.

During the late 1970s, enrollments in BS and MS programs in nursing increased. New associate degree (AD) programs were established, and graduates with only two years of post-high school training flocked to hospitals for well-paid jobs. Hospital positions for AD graduates were the same and paid the same as for nurses with BS degrees. This circumstance only increased the desire of BS graduates to pursue graduate education and specialty training.

Those two decades, the 1960s and 1970s, also saw significant growth in the development of doctoral education in nursing. PhD degrees, primarily in higher education and administration, were quickly followed by doctoral programs in theory development and testing. More recently, in the 1980s, programs in advanced practice research and in the theoretical underpinnings of practice were established. In the 1990s, programs of research in practice outcomes, effectiveness, and the relationship of practice to policy became the focus.

As the roles of the nurse practitioner and clinical specialist evolved in the 1970s, there was a bias toward the care setting—NPs practiced in the community with ambulatory patients, and clinical specialists were trained for inpatient care. This artificial barrier constrained the ability of advanced practice nurses to follow their patients across sites throughout an episode of illness. Today, those barriers are disappearing. Now, nurse practitioners work in institutions, and clinical specialists see their patients in outpatient settings. There is more responsibility for patients over time and across settings, and accountability is growing. Today's advanced practice nurses are empowered by nearly all state legislatures to prescribe medications, order laboratory and radiologic studies, and receive reimbursement for their services.

Surprisingly, these advancements have not further isolated nurses in independent roles, but instead have fostered their authoritative and complementary roles in team care with physicians.

With this rich background of professional development, which has been influenced partly by the social context of need, partly by the growth of biomedical knowledge, and partly by the economic and financial structure of the nation and its health care system, nursing has struggled for recognition, independence, and opportunity. Nursing is overshadowed by its partner, medicine, and many nursing services overlap with those of primary care physicians. Nursing thereby loses its fair portion of recognition for shared competencies. As for nursing's singular contributions—primarily in counseling, teaching, disease prevention, and health promotion—these are less riveting to the public and less clearly valuable than elegant technologies and highly visible life-and-death medical actions.

How can nursing shape its future to assure citizens of nurses' valuable and unique services? Nursing hopes to reach these goals in three ways: by advancing the educational preparation of its practitioners, by securing public recognition and access through demonstrated research, and by developing a structure in the nation's health care system that uses nursing services in a protected and focused way. Health care reform will shape the nursing profession in new ways during the last years of this century.

This book is intended to advise you about the value of graduate education in advancing your own career and to assist you in making the best selection of a graduate specialty. Whether your interests take you toward a primary care nurse practitioner career, toward the highly technical operating room team as a nurse anesthetist, or toward the detection, treatment, and counseling role of a psychiatric clinical specialist, you will be joining the profession at an advanced level with potential for a full scope of practice and direct decision making that never before has been possible.

Those of us who have been laboring in the vineyards these many decades are envious of your wonderful opportunities, grateful for having been part of the hard-won recognition for our practitioners, and proud to be your colleagues. Be all you can be, and make your decisions for advanced practice thoughtfully.

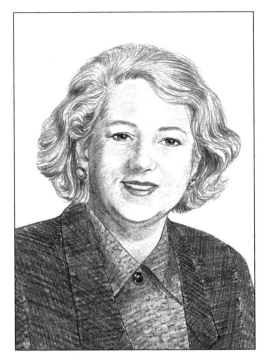

*Shirley Moore, PhD, RN,
is an assistant professor at Case Western
Reserve University School of Nursing,
in Cleveland, Ohio.*

Career Planning

Two days after I entered a diploma nursing school, the program was discontinued and we were told we'd be the last class to graduate. That was an early jolt of reality, and it made me realize that I had done less than a good job of researching my options and deciding where to get my training. It would be fair to say that I lacked a futuristic vision of my career.

Over the years I've worked hard to instill a forward-thinking attitude in nurses. In fact, most of my own career has been spent directing the development of nursing staff in large hospitals and other organizations. A significant part of that work required me to understand how nurses evolve in their work in order to help them enhance their careers.

After earning my diploma, I went on to get a BSN in 1974. Since then, I have earned two master's degrees, one in education and one in nursing, and in 1992 I got my PhD in nursing. Currently, I'm an assistant professor and teach nursing administration and am responsible for coordinating a joint MSN/MBA degree program. In that role, I counsel nurse executive students about career opportunities in nursing administration.

My philosophy as a career counselor is that instead of preparing themselves for a specific job, nurses should equip themselves with knowledge, skills, and experiences that will allow them flexibility and an opportunity to advance throughout their careers.

I start with two axioms. The first is that you must get — and remain — in touch with your personal needs and values. It's important to clarify your awareness of what you want out of life . . . and of the things you hope to avoid. In choosing career directions, nurses need to give careful consideration to practices that will accommodate their abilities, attitudes and lifestyles. What makes them feel comfortable at work? What makes them feel challenged? What gives them that little rush, that little thrill of self-fulfillment? Many people who come to me for counseling are simply having difficulty articulating and focusing on what they want. Often, all I need to do is help them begin thinking in the right direction.

After an initial exploratory conversation, I use questionnaires to help students identify their concerns and preferences — such issues as work hours, work environments, and social aspects of the job. Often these preferences can be determined through questions that have little to do with an actual job. For instance, whether a nurse would fare better working independently or on a team might be learned through such questions as, "Do you like going to parties?" and "Do you like talking on the telephone to friends?" A talent in written communication might be revealed by "Do you keep a diary?" These questions often are real eye-openers, and I'm always surprised at how important many nurses find the social aspects of work.

Students and entry-level nurses often are so busy that they forget about their personal needs. As a result, many find it difficult to evaluate their activities and their likes and dislikes. I try to make them feel comfortable examining and discussing the distasteful aspects. Once that is accomplished, we can talk about whether they should adjust to those shortcomings or consider a different type of activity. For instance, if a student hates confrontation, she might decide to take a class in interpersonal skills. An option would be to pursue independent practice.

My second axiom is that you must seek accurate information about yourself and the world of nursing. While you might believe you would be a great pediatrics nurse practitioner, you would be wise to ask others for their assessment before launching your career in that specialty. To get this appraisal, make a deal with your professors, peers, and clinicians with whom you have worked. The terms of the deal are that the person being asked for information agrees to give honest feedback in return for your promise to listen carefully and consider it as objectively as possible.

It is equally important to get information about the practicalities of nursing — how good is the job market and what credentials must you have to find a rewarding place in the profession? The fact is that nurses tend to be inexact about the credentials and experience required for any given position. Instead of considering what steps will lead to a desired goal, too many think loosely of the goal and have blind faith that if they put in enough time, they will reach it eventually. Obviously, this is not the most productive way to advance a career. I much prefer that students — especially those who hope to have advanced practices — carefully plan their education and work experiences. At a very basic level of such planning, know that some master's programs qualify students to sit for certification exams for specialty practice at the end. But some do not. If it's the same two years and the same money, you might as well choose the program that will increase your options. There is nothing wrong with using the tried-and-true method of listing the advantages and disadvantages of actions you are considering then making a choice after weighing them carefully.

It is essential for a young nurse to find a mentor — a professor ... a boss ... an established nurse — and follow that person around. Join the same organizations. Attend the same conferences, which usually include seminars on trends in the profession. Such exposure will lead to a long-term view of your career and will help prevent you from being overly concerned about the here and now of staff nursing.

Networking is no less important, and your skills in this activity should be honed throughout your professional life. A mentor can introduce you to important people. Never break those connections. Ask for business cards and pass out your own, quickly developing first-name relationships. Making friends with your peers is important, but you also must reach beyond your own level. Cultivate people who are where you want to be, and learn how they got there. You may be reluctant to bother the most notable nurses in your chosen field, but you will discover that most are quite approachable. And, this is a vital step because there is no substitute for personal relationships with nurses who are successfully doing with their lives what you intend to do with yours.

Few careers are founded on lucky breaks, so when talking to students, I emphasize the idea of investing — of strategically taking jobs just for the experience. It isn't necessary to stay forever; plan on staying for a reasonable period of time, say two years. On the other hand, if you have given a job a reasonable chance to be satisfying, don't stay on once you know it isn't working out. One of the reasons I encourage the development of a broad base of skills is that it enables nurses to switch jobs. Because they are able to move, they are free to admit they don't like something. Solid clinical skills plus a keen sense of self-awareness is the perfect formula for those who want to avoid feeling trapped in their jobs. If you gain those attributes, you will be able to sense career mistakes before they become crippling.

I encourage students I counsel to get a baccalaureate degree. Two-year programs offer a minimal level of education, and I have found that AD nurses often feel they don't have quite as much knowledge as they need. It is stressful to embark on a career for which you feel under-prepared, and it can lead to a great deal of insecurity in your work with patients. Students who do choose a two-year program should realize that their education qualifies them for little more than day-to-day care; strategic career management may have to be deferred. If your ambition is a broad role in nursing, but a two-year program is your only option at this time, you should consider developing a five-year plan to further your education.

When the time comes to advance your education, consider several factors when choosing a school. The school's reputation for quality is paramount. What do graduates and potential employers think of the school? What percentage of the school's graduates pass the state board exams? Does the school offer programs that address trends in the profession (eg, growing opportunities in community health and geriatric care)? Even if you don't intend to follow such trends, experience in those areas will probably serve you well. Because actual nursing experience, and plenty of it, is so desirable, select a school whose curriculum has a strong clinical component. That experience will be your trump card in those first job interviews.

Once you have a solid education, start building your career with fundamental experiences. New graduates should refine basic clinical and organizational skills in their first jobs. You may be tired of hearing the advice, "Do medical-surgical nursing for two years," but there is no better way to get those skills down pat. Besides, this is a good jumping-off point; starting in a more specialized area may make it harder to branch out later. In time, the clinical proficiency you gain in the beginning will free you to exercise your creative side in tailoring your care for individual patients.

As important as planning is, I believe it is possible to overplan. Remember, the world changes rapidly, and unknown configurations of health care, as well as new roles for nurses, are just over the horizon. If you enjoy your work at every level of your career, you will have planned well.

Once, nurses who wanted to advance their careers almost always moved into administrative duties. But that has been changing for some time. Today, nurses can advance to great rewards along clinical and entrepreneurial tracks as well. This will be more true tomorrow, and it should be a commanding factor in every nurse's career choice.

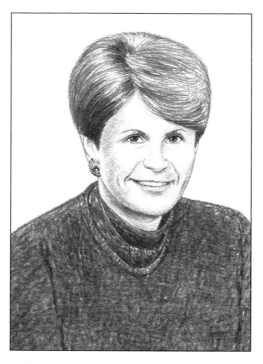

Colleen Conway-Welch, PhD, RN, CNM, FAAN,
is dean of the Vanderbilt University
School of Nursing,
Nashville, Tennessee.

Preparing for Advanced Practice

In the 1960s, when I chose nursing as a career, I thought I had made my final career decision. I didn't realize there were a hundred more educational and professional decisions still to come. Studies show that throughout their lifetimes, people embark on three different careers and change jobs seven times. Nursing offers enough flexibility to accommodate those changes and more.

I was attracted to nursing because it seemed to offer drama, a chance to travel, and the security of being able to support myself. After graduating from Georgetown in 1965 with my BSN and working as a staff nurse in Honolulu and San Francisco, I continued my academic studies at Catholic University, where I earned a master's degree in parent-child nursing. As part of that program, I took an elective course in nurse midwifery and subsequently became a certified nurse midwife. Finally, in 1973 I completed my PhD work in nursing at New York University. That background made it possible for me to alternate between service and educational positions, and currently I'm dean of the school of nursing at Vanderbilt University in Nashville. Our missions are teaching, practice, and research, and I've been involved in all of those areas. As my title suggests, I have had considerable experience in administration as well.

As this nation's health care system is reshaped, the opportunities for advanced practice nursing will increase and so will the responsibilities. Of course, with that expanding job market will come the need for a significant group of nurses with advanced clinical, case management, and administrative skills. While the profession will continue to provide jobs for AD and diploma-educated nurses, those nurses must understand that opportunities for advancement will depend increasingly on educational preparation. And because many educational avenues are open to nurses, it is essential that they be informed consumers.

Among U.S. nurses, about 60 percent hold associate degrees. Twenty-five percent are diploma graduates, and 15 percent have earned BSN degrees. Approximately five percent of the country's nurses have master's degrees and only one percent have doctorates. Choosing an appropriate educational program is the first essential career choice in nursing.

Young people considering a nursing career should give careful consideration to where they want to start and what they might want to be doing 10 years from now. In general, the professional opportunities associated with an AD or diploma program are similar: Graduates are qualified to work in community hospitals, long-term care facilities, and, in some cases, home care settings. BSN graduates have been prepared to work in community agencies, community hospitals and larger institutions, and home care. Initially, BSN graduates may not be given more responsibility than AD or diploma-graduate nurses, but because of their additional education, it's likely they will soon acquire increased authority and responsibility. Naturally, this varies from setting to setting. The AD nurse will have less autonomy in a tertiary care medical center than in a rural hospital, where the career opportunities might be more flexible, even without an additional degree.

Nursing students need a good sense of where they want to work directly after graduation and they should pursue an education that will open that first door. At the same time, it is important to consider what future doors an education will open. For instance, a BSN program offers students a broad education and prepares them to pursue a master's degree. So, if additional education is a goal, this probably is a wise choice. But choices also must be made with geography and finances in mind, and prospective nurses should not be discouraged from entering nursing simply because they are unable to enter a baccalaureate program. Still, I believe the nurse should someday return to school for a BSN if possible because the advantages a variety of liberal arts courses offer should not be underestimated.

Because of the structure of our health care system, nurses tend to expect more of themselves and to reach for responsibilities for which their education has not prepared them. Those who do this successfully earn salaries that are too low for the work being performed. Those who do it less well suffer stress as a result of the skewed relationship between their education and the responsibilities they are expected to discharge. Eventually, many nurses who find themselves in over their heads experience burnout. Proper preparation for advanced practice can alleviate these problems, and many hospitals are addressing this situation by offering tuition benefits to their nurses and requiring additional education for career advancement.

Advanced practice nursing is done by nurse practitioners (NP), clinical nurse specialists (CNS), certified nurse midwives (CNM), certified registered nurse anesthetists (CRNA), and nurse administrators.

Nurse practitioners are generally community based and have individual patients as clients. Some concentrate on primary care, including pediatric care, adult care, geriatric care, and women's health, while others care for adults and children as family nurse practitioners. The demand for nurse practitioners will increase, because they are extremely cost effective as primary care providers. While they need MD backup, they don't require the constant presence of a physician.

Indeed, research shows that 80 percent of the care primary care physicians provide can be handled by nurse practitioners. These nurses work according to protocols and can prescribe drugs. If a condition presents that is unusual or particularly complicated, they refer the patient to a physician.

One model for health care reform may result in having physicians focus on specialized care, while nurse practitioners assume responsibility for primary care. Primary care physicians would be available to the NP for problem cases. This is actually happening now with nurse practitioners who treat medically underserved populations in rural and inner-city areas. As nurses become more comfortable in these roles, new opportunities will present themselves in caring for the aging and chronically ill.

The tertiary care nurse practitioner reflects a new trend. Because the number of physician residency slots is declining in some hospitals, and because of restrictions on the hours residents can work, nurse practitioners are becoming viable alternatives to physicians for such duties as taking histories and performing physical examinations and certain diagnostic tests. No matter how any new health care reform may manifest itself, the emphasis will be on primary care, and nurse practitioners will be essential to its success.

While nurse practitioners work with individual patients, clinical nurse specialists serve as expert resources for other nurses and as role models for expert patient care and case management. Most clinical nurse specialists work in hospitals, but they also may be found in clinics and HMOs, long-term care facilities, and joint practices. As the title implies, a CNS has a particular clinical specialty, such as perinatal or adult health nursing. Further specialization is also possible, and an adult health CNS could refine his or her practice by subspecializing in oncology nursing. In addition to holding a graduate degree in a practice specialty, the CNS will be educated in other related areas, including advanced scientific concepts, research methodologies, and care management. Moreover, the clinical nurse specialist must be skilled in budgeting and case management. Certification by the appropriate national specialty organization is also required for the CNS.

The traditional definitions of a community-based nurse practitioner and a clinical nurse specialist are beginning to change as care settings cross all boundaries. As a result, the once-distinct lines between these specialties are blurring, because patients are hospitalized for shorter periods of time, and they're usually sicker when they go back to their communities. In accommodating to those changes, nurse practitioners are acquiring new skills in acute care, and clinical nurse specialists (who are being given added responsibility in the hospital) are refining their assessment skills. In this way, their areas of expertise are beginning to overlap.

Nursing administration is another option for nurses with master's degrees who have an interest in pursuing the required preceptorships in community health or in hospitals. Still other career options include practice as certified registered nurse anesthetists (who work in community or rural hospital settings) and as certified nurse midwives. As is the case with nurse practitioners, certified nurse midwives often practice among the underserved, but many are developing clienteles among well-educated, professional women who prefer the type of care a nurse midwife delivers.

Specialty certification by appropriate national organizations is an important educational step for nurses. While licensing indicates that a minimum amount of study sufficient to ensure safe nursing care has been completed, certification is achieved at the master's level and recognizes excellence. It reflects the completion of extra clinical work and demonstrates excellence in a particular specialty. Certification provides considerable prestige for the nurse — and considerable leverage in climbing the career ladder.

Opportunities at the doctorate level are wide open, because few nurses progress that far. Challenging positions for those who do are found in academia and research, and many who hold these degrees occupy high-level executive positions. A doctorate-prepared nurse in a research practice might work with staff nurses and clinical nurse specialists to define problems in patient care and identify ways of making care more cost efficient with better patient outcomes. While a researcher might be indirectly involved with the care of an unusual patient for investigative purposes, this kind of nurse is more likely to concentrate on studying selected patient populations and analyzing trends in patient care.

Three avenues are available to nurses who want to pursue doctoral education. The two most common are the doctorate of science in nursing (DSN), which is a professional degree that emphasizes clinical practice, and the PhD in nursing, which is primarily oriented toward research. The nursing doctorate (ND) is another professional degree that may replace the DSN in the future. The advent of the ND is the result of efforts to model nursing on other practice disciplines. For example, physicians and lawyers must earn undergraduate degrees before entering their professional programs. An ND program is similarly structured and requires a baccalaureate degree, not necessarily in nursing, for entry. Eventually, this may become the primary pathway to professional nursing practice at the advanced-practice level.

Today, doctoral nurses are rare, but our profession is encouraging younger students to consider advanced education. By the time nurses reach their 30s and 40s, they grow more receptive to the idea of continuing their studies, but at this stage they also have other demands on their lives. We acknowledge the fact that advanced-level nursing offers more accountability, more opportunity, more responsibility, and, of course, more money.

Case management is becoming a focal point in all areas of advanced practice. This is a method of managing the patient's contact with the health care system by helping him interpret his needs and serving as his advocate within the system. To a limited degree, nurses have always done that, but now it's becoming a recognized function, and it is being translated into specific, formal training.

A primary function of nursing is to diagnose and treat common health problems, but there's been some controversy over the word *diagnosis* because it implies a medical decision. However, diagnosing is simply a process of critical thinking, and advanced practice gives the nurse a chance to do that in greater depth.

While we in the nursing profession strive to keep nurses employed in nursing, it must be noted that nursing is an excellent background for other positions in the health care industry, and many nurses are employed throughout this area.

As nurses' roles change, so do the education programs that make career advancement possible. For example, nursing curricula are beginning to address contemporary issues in budgeting and cost management as well as negotiation and delegation. In this era of careful economy, these are essential skills that will enable nurses to participate in managing the costs of care. In this fashion, nursing schools are becoming more responsive than ever before to the needs of students. We're seeing more competency-based learning and more adaptation to individual learning styles. We're also seeing a greater use of technology, especially in computer-aided instruction.

Nontraditional nursing programs, such as the one at Vanderbilt, are becoming more popular. Here, we require students to complete three years of college before entering the nursing program. Then, they spend a calendar year taking basic nursing courses, followed by another year in a specialty master's program. They bypass the baccalaureate, but earn their master's degree in two years. In addition, to strengthen the practice component of a nurse's education, we've opened a primary care clinic and plan to open four or five more. All will be managed by nurse practitioners. Those clinics move us out of the academic ivory tower and into the trenches.

Flexibility is increasingly the hallmark of nursing education in the United States. Many schools now offer post-master's options that allow a master's-prepared nurse in one specialty area to take additional course work and change direction to a new career specialty. This also enables nurses to obtain certification in other nursing specialties. I believe that as practice and other career opportunities expand — and as additional educational avenues are opened — nurses should be, and will be, encouraged to explore new opportunities in nursing.

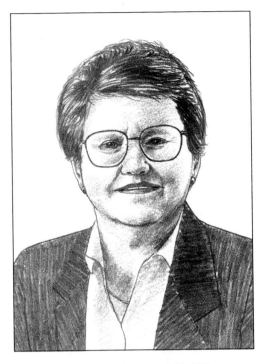

Karen S. O'Connor, MA, RN,
is director of practice, economics, and policy
for the American Nurses Association,
Washington, D.C.

Ethics, Standards, Regulations

Nursing practice is guided by a humanistic philosophy that recognizes the value of each individual. To a degree that is unique, human beings are able to reflect, create, and communicate. Once refined by education, this aptitude allows us to make self-directed choices and take deliberate action in shaping our lives. Respect for this potential is the source of all human values and rights. It is the basis of every goal for which we strive as nurses.

I chose nursing as a profession because of my desire to help people. The nature of my abilities resulted in a career in which the help I provide takes place some distance from the bedside, in efforts to increase opportunity and improve working conditions for nurses, to improve the quality of and access to health care, and to advance the way our profession addresses its responsibilities.

The practice of nursing arises from a traditional ethos of service — of protecting and regenerating health, of nurturing the sick and comforting the dying. Many state nursing practice acts and the preamble to the American Nurses Association *Code for Nurses* use a contemporary definition of this creed, defining nursing as "the diagnosis and treatment of human responses to actual or potential health problems." These responses, whether physical, emotional, or cognitive, are distinct from the health problem itself, which usually is the object of well-defined health care interventions. Complex human responses are nursing's focus and involve the whole person at multiple levels of functioning. As a result, the approach we take in providing help must be deliberately holistic, considering the client's needs in a human context rather than in a biomedical context.

Human responses to health problems are so varied that it is difficult to categorize them discretely. This array of responses requires great sensitivity on the nurse's part. Some patients must cope with extreme pain, others with limitations in the ability to care for themselves. Illness and treatment may produce emotions in the form of fear, anxiety, loneliness, or grief. Health changes may require difficult adjustments in self-image and may exacerbate problems in relationships. The ability to make decisions or personal choices may be impaired.

This is difficult terrain. As nurses, we believe that the best way to achieve high quality in the services we deliver is to adhere to the values, behaviors, and nursing interventions that constitute effective practice. To maximize the profession's ability to meet human needs in a productive manner, the American Nurses Association with its constituent state nurses associations has established a code of ethics, defined standards of nursing practice, and influenced the development of state nurse practice acts that establish the qualifications for practice. Standards require continuing attention to ensure that they reflect current vision and advances in knowledge and technology. A primary goal of the ANA is to provide support and guidance that will help individual practitioners to perform their duties. Another is to help the profession respond to changes in the health care environment by articulating practice components in a way that makes it possible to evaluate our services in terms of patient outcomes.

Nursing has evolved to meet the changing human needs of society. Indeed, our profession has a strong identity as consumer advocates, and the internalization of ethical values is fundamental to our history and to the attainment of our contemporary objectives. Thus, the regulation of nursing's relationship to society is, to a large degree, initiated within the profession. While it is necessary to protect the public from unqualified and unsafe practitioners, there are clear relationships between highly restrictive legislation imposed by persons outside the profession, and a curtailment in the innovation and growth of nursing practice and in public access to specialized nursing services. The most effective balance is reached when basic competency requirements are set by law and professional associations maintain higher standards.

Self-regulation begins with practitioners. In becoming nurses, each of us makes a moral commitment to uphold *The Code for Nurses,* which outlines the profession's values and goals. Adopted by the American Nurses Association in 1950, these principles are the ethical foundation of nursing practice, from which all other standards and regulations arise.

Reflecting the priorities expressed in the code, *Standards of Clinical Nursing Practice* are authoritative statements that describe the responsibilities for which all practitioners are held accountable in their relationship with all clients. These standards articulate the procedures and performance that comprise the nursing process, providing not only a structure for practice, but a method of evaluating practice.

The regulation and control of nursing practice by the profession means that individual nurses are accountable for the quality of their practice and for the care received by clients. Neither an employer's policies nor a physician's orders waive our responsibility. This accountability is legally binding, and nurses may be named as defendants in malpractice cases. Violations of the social contract between nursing and society reflect on every nurse. Adherence to the ethics and standards of practice is enforced within the profession. Violations are addressed through peer review.

Health care today is technical and complex, and lawmakers must rely significantly on the profession in setting legal qualifications that authorize a nurse to practice. In fact, the American Nurses Association periodically issues proposed revisions to state legislation that affects nursing practice. These are intended to bring important issues to the attention of policymakers and to facilitate legislation that reflects advances in the profession while protecting the public.

Regulations associated with state nurse practice acts are implemented through state-appointed nursing boards that consist of registered professional nurses — usually recommended by the state professional association — and members of the public. While specifics of these acts vary among states, they define the minimum level of competence required to ensure reasonable protection of the public's health, safety, and welfare. This level of competence is attained and sustained in accredited institutions in accordance with stipulated educational requirements. It is measured via standardized licensing examinations. And it is enforced through means that include a definition and regulation of the functions and procedures performed in nursing practice, as generally are established through statements issued by the ANA and through discipline in the form of reprimand or suspension, revocation, or denial of a license to practice.

The Code for Nurses and Standards of Clinical Nursing Practice, as well as licensure laws and regulations associated with state nurse practice acts are interrelated and, at times, overlapping guidance systems that support each other. Although each may differ in its purpose and methods, together they set practice definitions that allow nurses to discharge their responsibilities in a way that is consistent with a moral commitment to the profession and high-quality nursing care. Such delineations enable other health care professionals and society as a whole to measure the degree to which the nursing profession has lived up to expectations.

Ultimately, the caliber of nursing care is conditioned by factors that cannot be mandated through legislation or practice standards. This is true because, in addition to clinical and technical expertise, effective nursing practice requires considerable skills in judgement and interpersonal relations.

The Code for Nurses with Interpretive Statements is a basic guide. It delineates a structure of ethically responsible conduct applicable to a broad variety of circumstances. By identifying troubling issues, ruling out inappropriate actions, and helping the individual make the necessary transition from personal to professional values, it offers guidance for executing the nurse's professional role.

In every interaction between human beings, an astonishing amount of nonverbal information is exchanged. Voice tone and modulation, facial expression and body postures, and other factors too subtle to be deliberately controlled govern the quality of human communication. Indeed, the information transmitted through nonverbal behavior can be far more significant than the spoken word. Consequently, whether articulated or left unspoken, a nurse's values and attitudes and their influence on the client have a significant impact on the quality of nursing care.

Attitudinal elements exert influence on every aspect of nursing — the services we perform, our relationships with patients and their families and other members of the health care team, and the public's perception of our profession. Human response is a dynamic process that can be difficult to anticipate. By studying *The Code for Nurses with Interpretive Statements* and examining situations in its light until we have made it part of ourselves, its principles will begin reflexively to shape our behavior. In my own case, the ethical code for nurses has become an aspect of the broader ethic that governs my relationship with the world. There is no contradiction between my professional values and those which guide my personal interactions. Any discord between these realms would impair my professional performance and subject me to uncomfortable inner conflict.

The socialization that enables us to function effectively as professionals is a continuous process of influence and assimilation. It involves not only acquiring knowledge and skills, but also developing the habits, attitudes, and motivations that give rise to a sense of professional identity. Assimilating nursing's ethical values is no less important than acquiring clinical expertise.

The Code for Nurses expresses nursing's conscience and is designed to accommodate diversity within the profession and within the populations we serve. Its stated principles are not negotiable: When individuals become nurses, they make a moral commitment to act in accordance with the profession's ethics. Professional ethics do not represent an isolated position or a general wish to do the right thing. Instead they form a set of comprehensive and cohesive principles that serve as a guide for determining appropriate attitudes and conduct. Our code of ethics does not promise infallibility. Nor does it guarantee easy answers.

If my ethical principles are in conflict with a specific intervention, I have the right to refuse to participate — if, and only if, other arrangements can be made for the client's care. If I feel that I lack the competence to perform a specific procedure, I must refuse to do it and find someone who is qualified. If I am called upon to make an ethical decision and it is beyond my capacity to do so, it is my obligation to consult with someone who can help me in that judgement.

Self-interest is never an acceptable reason for refusing a responsibility. As a nurse, it is my obligation periodically to review the code and evaluate my own practice in relationship to its principles. The code is best used when considered in relation to an individual's personal assumptions and understanding.

The first tenet of *The Code for Nurses* is that the nurse provides services with respect for human dignity and the individuality of the client, unrestricted by considerations of social or economic status, personal attributes, or the nature of health problems. Because clients make the ultimate choices about their own well-being, the primary goal of our actions must be to sustain and strengthen their ability for conscious self-determination, which defines the quality of humanity. The preservation of autonomy and dignity under even the most demanding circumstances is essential for individuals to maintain their self-respect.

One of the most difficult things for all of us to accept, I believe, is that a client's view of the world may be very different from our own. If we glimpse this different vision, we often think it is wrong, that the client's humanity thus has less value and that the client's choices are thus wrong. A part of nursing's function is to provide education and guidance toward greater well-being. Yet, as professionals we must make a careful distinction between a client's actions that result from emotional confusion or lack of information and those prompted by a philosophical or cultural stance that is merely different from our own. Individual autonomy is a central principle of *The Code for Nurses*.

I believe that a moral truth is based on firm conviction rather than empirical evidence. Science has no absolute answers for ethical and philosophical issues, but this makes them no less valid. The result of an action is not directly the concern; what one feels about the result is more important. Such issues can only be addressed by examined thought and consensus values (which may be mandated as law, regulation, standard) and through individual conviction that arises from a balance of personal experience and a cultural context that may stretch back for centuries.

The respect nursing holds for human dignity and our efforts to support the autonomy of individuals includes a commitment to action that benefits and protects the client. This is a commitment to truth that allows each client's responses, deliberations, and choices to be based on information that, even if painful, is accurate and complete. It is a commitment to confidentiality that does not betray our intimate relationship with clients; to fidelity in the promises we make; and to justice that acknowledges every individual's humanity and worth.

The primacy of the value contemporary nursing places upon independence has a strong relationship to our cultural heritage as Americans. For many of us, autonomy is worth more than comfort or safety, and we must offer this choice to our clients.

The independence nursing supports for its clients is equally necessary to the profession itself. In order to provide high-quality consistent care while maintaining the ability to respond to changing social needs, the nursing profession must control the designation and performance of professional services, the physical and psychological environment in which services are delivered, and the philosophical premises determining these service and environment factors. To the degree that any of these interrelated elements are controlled by external agencies, the potential for sensitive response to needs is diminished, and our care becomes subject to inconsistency.

The professional values that orient each nurse to the community of need rather than self-interest and the commitment to uphold those values provide the basis of nursing's strength. Our society has acknowledged its trust in support of nursing's autonomy. Now, it is the responsibility of each of us, as nurses and as individuals, to work for the goal of self-regulation and to advance our efforts to protect, support, and enhance the well-being of everyone we serve.

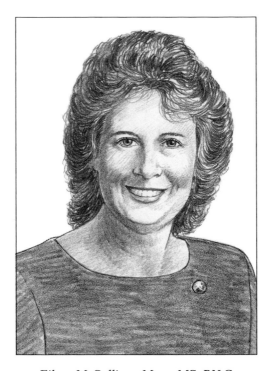

Eileen M. Sullivan-Marx, MS, RN,C,
is an adult nurse practitioner who
specializes in geriatrics.
She is project manager for the
Collaborative Assessment and Rehabilitation
for Elders Program, and a doctoral candidate
at the University of Pennsylvania
School of Nursing,
Philadelphia, Pennsylvania.

On the Horizon: Direct Reimbursement

Health care administrators, practicing physicians, and third-party reimbursers readily admit that nurses are indispensable in the vast majority of inpatient and outpatient care practices. Nurses provide some of the most advanced and intensive health care services available, and we are essential to the health care system. Unfortunately for most of us, we also are invisible. That is, we are invisible when it comes to the patient's bill or a third-party reimburser's payment statement. But if current trends are any indication, the services nurses provide will soon be recognized from a reimbursement perspective. The results will have implications for virtually every practicing nurse in the country.

The idea that nurses should be reimbursed directly is not new. In fact, as long ago as 1948, the American Nurses Association (ANA) formally advocated that nurses be eligible for third-party payments. Throughout the 1950s, 1960s, and 1970s, other directives and statements calling for (1) inclusion of nursing services as a benefit in prepaid health plans and (2) direct remuneration for services were issued by the ANA and other nursing associations. However, real progress in this area did not come until the late 1970s, when the state of Washington, as a result of strong lobbying efforts by nurses, passed legislation that permitted advanced practice nurses to receive direct payment from private insurers and other reimbursers. Throughout the 1980s, other states followed suit, virtually all as a result of nurse advocacy. Today 25 states permit advanced practice nurses to be paid directly by insurers and Medicaid. Some sections of Medicare laws have changed as well.

Why, after years of resistance, did these changes finally begin to occur? The answer will help explain why today's health care environment is ripe for empowering all nurses to receive the benefits of direct reimbursement.

In the late 1970s, when advanced practice nurses began pushing for direct reimbursement, two important things were happening. One is that nursing was experiencing a kind of professional revolution. Other health care providers were beginning to acknowledge that nurses are more than servants to physicians. We were being better trained, we were becoming more specialized, and we were performing more and more complex procedures. In general, as the value of nurses went up, so did their financial rewards. In part, this was a result of a dramatic nursing shortage that developed as an increasing number of nurses chose not to practice. Hospitals in particular could not afford vacancies in nursing positions, because such vacancies affected the quality of patient care as well as institutional accreditation.

Another significant feature of that period is that nurse practitioners were increasing in numbers and assuming more responsibilities. In fact, in some settings, nurse practitioners had begun to perform duties that once had been solely within the domain of physicians. These nurses were indispensable. And yet, if anyone took time to measure the business (and subsequent reimbursement) they generated against the salaries they were paid, it was obvious that nurses were not getting their fair share. Indeed, their services, which were so essential in the operation of most facilities, never even appeared on the bill. Reimbursement went to the physician or to the hospital itself. This was true despite the fact that nurse practitioners were more cost effective and not cost inflationary.

In time, many nurse practitioners decided they had had enough. They wanted to change the way they were getting paid, but their discontent had to do with more than money. They wanted to be recognized for their professionalism. Nurses could call themselves professionals, but the term was meaningless unless they were considered professional colleagues by physicians, administrators, reimbursers, and others outside of nursing. The challenge, then, was to make it apparent that what nurses did in their practices was intrinsically valuable. Through diligent efforts at education — achieved mainly through professional associations — more and more advanced practice nurses have been able to convince their state legislators that it is in society's best interest to reimburse nurses for their services.

When I became interested in direct reimbursement, I was working as a nurse practitioner in Pennsylvania. It took me six months to understand how the system worked. It took even longer to work with other nurses to develop a task force through my state association to address the problem. The task force provided information and education to legislators, insurers, and other policy makers, but only after five years of intense work on our part were laws changed to permit direct payment.

Today, 25 states mandate that Medicaid and private insurers must give advanced practice nurses the opportunity to receive direct payment for their care and services. These nurses have a choice: They can opt for the direct payment, or they can work for a salary. Consequently, they are free to design practices that provide unprecedented financial opportunities and career flexibility. This mandate also gives nurses who wish to remain in salaried positions considerable leverage in negotiation for better pay or benefits.

Still, the system is not yet equitable; 25 states do not permit direct reimbursement for nurses. Moreover, changes at the federal level have been piecemeal. For example, the government allocates Medicaid funds to each state, provides a framework of services for which this money can be used, and lets individual states handle disbursement. Currently, 38 states permit nurses to receive direct Medicaid reimbursement. And regulations are in place that will do the same in 11 other states. It is a different story with Medicare.

Medicare payments come directly from the federal government; so do the regulations on who may receive these payments. Medicare laws now allow direct reimbursement to certified nurse midwives and nurse anesthetists and to nurse practitioners who practice in designated rural areas. The lack of direct payment for other services is a product of today's climate at the federal level, specifically at the Health Care Financing Administration (HCFA). HCFA's emphasis on cost containment has created the perception that extending direct reimbursement to another category of provider would be inflationary. This perception prevails despite the fact that several states and private reimbursers consider direct payment to nurses to be cost effective, and research supports this view.

What bearing does direct reimbursement have on nurses who are not in advanced practices? Quite a bit, actually.

Most nurses are salaried or receive hourly rates of pay from their employers. Though this system has its advantages and is preferred by many nurses, it is important to remember that money for salaries or hourly payments comes from outside of the institution, while the salary levels are set inside the institution. Ideally, the pay should be based on the type of services delivered, the demand for nurses in that practice type and in the surrounding geographical area, and the individual nurse's experience. In essence, it should reflect supply and demand — which is not a bad system until one considers that most other high-level health care professionals receive payment based on both supply and demand *and* services rendered. The latter factor is a result of training and experience and expertise, and it may be the most important component of the reimbursement formula.

The pay scale for nurses has not traditionally been based on an evaluation of their services; what we do has never been quantified in a formal way. This is very different from physicians, whose services are broken down not only by specialties, but by procedures within those specialties. It is also different from allied health professionals (eg, physical and occupational therapists) who work in selected areas and perform specific — and thus reimbursable — tasks. Nurses in hospitals regularly perform services, such as starting intravenous lines and monitoring electrocardiograms, for which physicians charge insurers.

In part, nursing services were never quantified because of the way the profession has evolved over the last 30 years. As technology advanced and the practices of physicians became increasingly special-ized, nurses responded by filling in gaps in patient care. The pro-fession was glad to accept the responsibility, and the training and education of nurses became even more sophisticated. Today, we routinely perform advanced procedures that, had they existed 30 years ago, would have been entrusted only to a physician. In fact, over the last decade, many teaching hospitals have begun considering the utilization of advanced practice nurses to meet service needs as the number of medical residents decreases. Many of the services these physicians once delivered (eg, admissions evaluations, postoperative services, discharge planning, and even coordination of postdischarge services) are being taken up by staff nurses and advanced practice nurses. Everything has changed — except the way we are paid.

Now more than ever before, nurses need to understand that what they are doing for an institution generates revenues. Even if they are paid by salary, quantification of their services is essential for recog-nition. Quantification also can be a negotiation tool for career advancement. For example, nursing services have a direct impact on length of stay, a factor that has extreme importance in every hospital. This is true because most insurers reimburse hospitals according to a patient's diagnosis-related group, regardless of how long the patient is hospitalized. Increasingly, it is nursing's province to make sure that patients follow their care plans and are discharged in a timely manner. This includes evaluating the need for postdischarge care and serving as liaison with other health care professionals and social workers to ensure that services are provided on schedule. This coordination is essential, because patients who are discharged early need more care at home. Nurses also counsel family members and teach them to care for the patient. All of these valuable activities take place in addition to bedside care.

In the outpatient setting, nurses often perform basic health evalua-tions and deliver preventive care. Data collected in states where nurses do receive direct payment from reimbursers show that this care is cost effective and highly efficacious.

The push for health care reform in the current administration is highly supportive of nursing's position on reimbursement. It is hoped that part of the health care package that eventually is recommended will eliminate the regulatory barriers to nurse reimbursement that now exist at state and federal levels.

No matter what direction health care takes in the future, nurses will serve as their own best champions by striving for greater recognition. The best way to do this is by working through our professional associ-ations to gather information about what services nurses perform and how much these services cost. The more data we compile, the better case we will be able to make for direct reimbursement. And the greater control we will be able to exert over our own professional careers.

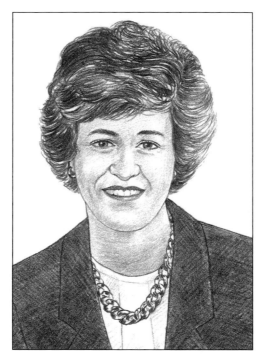

Sue Thomas Hegyvary, PhD, RN, FAAN,
is dean and professor at the
University of Washington School of Nursing
Seattle, Washington.

Home Care

Many of the nursing greats in the past century focused their efforts on caring for people at home. This area of nursing practice has changed dramatically, yet it retains the essential values and principles of nursing and will be an increasingly important field of practice in the future. This and other community-based services will grow in importance as the American health care system is transformed. This brief paper gives an overview of this important component of the health care system.

At the beginning of this century, virtually all medical and nursing care was provided in people's homes. In many situations, especially for the care associated with childbirth or care for the chronically ill, nurses actually lived with patients' families for extended periods of time. At that time, the average life expectancy in the United States was 47 years. Most deaths occurred at home.

In the early decades of the twentieth century, hospitals were considered institutions of last resort, and they mainly served the less fortunate in our society. While the industrial revolution was changing the face of American business and industry, technological changes were slower to come in health care. However, our understanding of disease-causing organisms was growing rapidly, and so was our understanding of what treatments could eradicate them. Those discoveries brought technology into the hospital.

As that change occurred, hospitals came to be recognized as the best places to go for health care services. Then, to some degree, and now to a large degree, the problems associated with the centrality of hospitals in our health care system pertain to costs and to the fact that there often is greater emphasis on the provider than on the patient. Even so, there is no question that the successes of care and treatment in both public health and hospitals changed our lives. One indicator of such success is that our average life expectancy is now in the seventh decade. And most deaths no longer occur at home, but in hospitals — in the care of strangers.

During decades of emphasis on treating patients in hospitals, home care and community health nursing have remained important areas of practice. Nurses today no longer live in their patients' homes, but they do make home visits to assess health status, give medical treatments, provide counseling about health, and make referrals for community services. In general, they promote recovery from illnesses and help those they care for adapt to life with chronic illness.

Sometimes, they have the sad task of helping a patient and family face impending death.

A major change in the emphasis on home care services occurred in the 1980s, not only because the importance of these services was recognized, but also because of changes in reimbursement policies for hospital care. Indeed, most people are hospitalized simply because they require continuous nursing care. This is a costly means of providing such care, so cost-containment efforts targeted reductions in length of stay.

Cost-containment efforts led to what has been called the quicker-and-sicker approach to hospitalization, in which patients are discharged more quickly and more in need of further care than ever before. Now, for example, preoperative work-ups are completed before admission, and even patients who will undergo very serious operations are admitted on the day of surgery. After early discharge, such patients depend on the delivery of highly complex home care.

Increasingly, referrals for nursing services in the home are made by primary care practitioners or other community-based providers. This approach often makes it possible for patients to avoid hospitalization.

A home care practice incorporates the best of nursing traditions and values. It focuses on the health of individuals and families in the context of their own homes. It also provides to nurses the challenge of applying their knowledge and skills in an autonomous fashion. Home care nurses are directly involved in managing their patients' illnesses, and they employ a growing variety of highly technical skills. In addition, the community context challenges home care nurses to consider the relationship of health and illness to numerous other factors, including nutrition, education, ethnicity, stress, and other social and environmental variables.

This range of abilities is developed through a broad base of education. As the complexity of home care services continues to increase, this advanced practice specialty will require graduate-level education. And even though most nurses currently in the field do not have graduate degrees, today's students and new graduates would be well served by advanced degrees.

I challenge nursing graduates to consider community nursing and, particularly, care in the home as an uncommonly rewarding career. This specialty offers a view of life that encompasses patient, family, and community in the broader societal context. That's where nursing started, and for all the evolution that has occurred in the delivery of health care, it remains the heart and soul of nursing.

Occupational Health

Kay M. Arendasky, MSN, RN, CRNP,
is an occupational health services consultant,
and program coordinator of the occupational health graduate
program at the University of Pennsylvania
School of Nursing.

Whether an employee smokes or uses seat belts isn't the kind of issue one usually associates with occupational health nursing. But this field has changed dramatically during the last 20 years, and now an employee's lifestyle choices have become as integral a part of occupational health as safe working conditions.

Spiraling health care costs have shown employers that occupational health services are cost effective. If they can prevent work-related injuries and illnesses and help employees stay generally healthier, these services reduce both workers' compensation costs and general medical liability. After all, a single premature baby can consume a million dollars in medical resources. Unfortunately, most companies become interested in occupational health services only after the company president has his first heart attack.

As companies look for ways to manage the cost of providing health care coverage to employees, the demand for occupational health nurses, particularly nurse practitioners, is mushrooming. And because the field addresses direct patient care as well as prevention and health promotion, it's the perfect place for a nurse practitioner. I maintain a private practice and am program coordinator for the occupational health graduate program at the University of Pennsylvania.

It used to be that practically every occupational health care provider had gray hair. As a result, the field developed a reputation for being a place where doctors and nurses could retire; it was a way to give up the grind of an independent practice and get regular hours. And because it was an "industry job," there was a perception that occupational health nursing was management-driven, with little real concern for workers. Indeed, many companies used to view occupational health as a legal mandate rather than good business. They believed they were complying with a regulation, not offering a service; they believed they were spending money, not achieving long-term economies.

Although the United States once had huge immigrant populations that provided an almost limitless labor force, that's no longer the case. Companies now understand that recruiting and training people cost money, and that high turnover wastes it. Now, they want to find ways to keep employees, and occupational health nurses are are able to help them do that. In addition, the establishment in 1970 of the Occupational Safety and Health Administration (OSHA) meant a quantum leap forward for workers' rights and for legitimizing the profession of occupational health. As OSHA established standards, the need for occupational health professionals — and industrial hygienists and safety personnel — grew.

Because occupational health nurses usually are the only health care professionals in a particular corporate setting, their expertise is taken for granted. Consequently, the nurse establishes policies and procedures, identifies and prevents hazardous conditions, provides direct care to and acts as a case manager for workers. The nurse is concerned with the epidemiology of work-related injuries and illnesses. If several employees present with similar problems, the challenge is to identify the cause.

Take as an example warehouse workers who must lift boxes from a pallet and place them on a conveyor belt. If the employees work only on one side of the conveyor, they may be headed for repetitive motion problems. The nurse might suggest that instead of repeating the same activity for 40 hours a week, the workers should be rotated off the line and into a job that uses another muscle group. At least, the workers could move periodically to the other side of the conveyor belt.

Other workplace hazards are more complex. If exposure to dangerous chemicals is a problem, the nurse might work with management to substitute an innocuous substance, or to reduce exposure by improving ventilation systems or installing hoods that protect the worker. It may be enough to provide personal masks and gloves or other protective clothing, but because such measures depend on compliance, the nurse may decide they are inappropriate.

The occupational health nurse is concerned with policies and procedures that may affect workers' health. For instance, what is the policy for requiring health examinations before assigning an employee to a job? Is the examination stringent enough to protect the worker and the company? If a job-related injury or illness occurs, what is the procedure for reporting it? How does the company respond in such cases: Are there guidelines for determining whether the employee should continue working, be sent home, or be taken to the hospital? The nurse may be responsible for setting such parameters. In addition to these duties, the nurse may review the company's human resource policies, offering advice about adherence to OSHA regulations and even helping set policies for hiring new employees.

In many companies, occupational nurses provide general health care, treating such ailments as earaches, stomachaches and sore throats. Some conduct tests for blood pressure, blood sugar, and cholesterol and organize seminars for CPR or smoking cessation.

These activities create a healthier work force and increase productivity by reducing the number of lost man hours. Another significant benefit should be a reduction in insurance costs. In fact, occupational health nurses are increasingly being used to extend health care to employees' families. One thing is certain: Occupational nursing is making health care available to millions of blue collar workers who would otherwise have no access to care.

Teaching is a big part of the job. For instance, people who use computers extensively need to change their work habits periodically in order to work more safely. For warehouse workers, the nurse might sponsor a seminar on how to avoid injury when lifting heavy items. Conducting seminars on substance abuse and emotional illness is a logical activity for the occupational health nurse.

To be a successful occupational nurse, you need the skills of a salesperson, because you will have to market yourself and your services. This is especially true if you're talking about health care and your employer is thinking about dollars. So, instead of breaking the news that a new ventilation system to control exposure to hazardous vapors will cost $25,000, the more effective nurse might say that an investment of $25,000 will save hundreds of thousands of dollars in medical claims and lost hours.

Most nurses are accustomed to having support from a wide range of other health care professionals. However, that support is not likely to be found in a corporate setting, and assessment and diagnostic skills assume paramount importance. As a result, my students — whether they are on a clinical or administrative track — take courses in toxicology, industrial hygiene, and industrial safety. One course will not make you an expert, but it may instill an awareness of significant issues. And because injuries are common in industry, knowledge of emergency care is a requirement for occupational nurses.

Beyond a strong clinical foundation and an independent nature, nurses in industry are well served by a combination of business acumen and street smarts, and they must be able to handle confrontations. They also must be able to work in front of an audience because few incidents attract more attention than a workplace injury. In the hospital, only hospital personnel see you work. In occupational health, the entire work force may be watching.

Occupational health nurses have three categories of clients: the individual employee, the aggregate group of employees, and the employer. The needs of those clients occasionally conflict, so it's up to the nurse to find an equitable balance. While workers once resented occupational health professionals as representatives of management, I think that has changed. Now, in most settings, we're seen as legitimate advocates for the worker.

Working in occupational health is not unlike belonging to a religious order; you must commit to the higher authority of ethical considerations. You surely must not countenance unsafe working conditions — or the employer's refusal to correct them — simply for the sake of a paycheck.

Rather than working as full-time employees for corporate employers, some occupational nurses hire themselves out on a contract basis, or work at local health care facilities used by workers whose companies don't have their own nursing staff. Many companies believe that contracting with independent nurses gives them flexibility. Another option is to work as a consultant, perhaps for an insurance company, advising its clients on occupational health issues.

More now than ever before, companies are realizing that providing quality occupational health nursing is smart business. Regulatory shifts in workers' compensation and rising costs of medical benefits have made clear the importance of protecting the health of employees. And some managed care providers offer significant discounts to companies with occupational health services. For nurses, the result is a fledgling field where they can assume great responsibility. The notion that employment in this field is a form of retirement no longer has validity. Instead, the delivery of top-quality occupational health care depends on nurses with a true commitment to the well-being of workers. Tomorrow's challenge is to create a network of primary care in the workplace. But for now, we're getting the attention of corporations before their top executives have heart attacks.

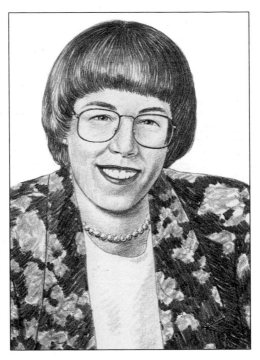

*Barbara J. Daly, MSN, MA, RN, FAAN,
is assistant professor at Case Western
Reserve University School of Nursing
in Cleveland, Ohio.
She also is assistant professor in the
School of Medicine, and assistant director of
nursing at University Hospitals of Cleveland.*

Blended Roles

Nursing not only allows me to do the things I enjoy, it has given me three careers in one. I work in a clinical practice that I created myself, I am a primary investigator in a groundbreaking research project, and I teach what I have learned to graduate and undergraduate students. Where else in health care could one find such an opportunity for flexibility and creativity?

In 1969, I received my bachelor's degree in nursing and began practicing at Cleveland's University Hospitals, which is associated with Case Western Reserve University. I have stayed for more than 20 years because both the hospital and the university provide excellent environments for professional growth.

During my first four years in nursing, I worked as a psychiatric nurse and a medical-surgical nurse before beginning work in critical care. Throughout this period, I studied part time for my master's degree in nursing, completing it in 1972. Soon after, I accepted a head nurse position in the intensive care unit (ICU) and began teaching graduate students at Case Western. I didn't know it at the time, but these new management and teaching responsibilities would eventually lead me into a new clinical practice and serve as the foundation for an advanced research project.

As a head nurse, I managed the ICU, supervising personnel and scheduling work loads for the staff nurses. Many of our patients were critically ill, and I participated directly in their care. At that time, advanced medical technology enabled us to save patients who surely would have died a few years earlier. But our successes often involved trade-offs — cases in which the patient's quality of life was seriously compromised.

The new technology was capable of saving lives, but it began to raise questions for me. What does the nurse do if a patient refuses to accept our sophisticated care? Does a patient's desire to die take precedence over our ability to prevent death? What is the nurse's position if a patient has issued a do-not-resuscitate order but the family wants it rescinded? Our education has prepared us to give the best possible care, but what do we do if the patient doesn't want it? These were serious dilemmas, and there were no guidelines for answering them. The circumstances were just too new.

For a while, I kept my thoughts to myself. But soon, staff nurses began approaching me with the same concerns. It was clear that technology would continue advancing, and questions of this nature —

ethical questions — would continue shadowing its progress. I decided that the only way to find some resolution to them was to examine what had been said through the ages about ethics, morality, and the courses of action affecting life and death. This meant going back to school in order to study philosophy and ethics.

When people confront issues for which there are no clear answers, the decisions they make often seem to be very subjective judgement calls. It was reassuring to learn that philosophy offers a precise and logical way to examine questions and arrive at answers. The study of philosophy reveals guidelines for sorting out issues, identifying relevant factors, and learning which are the most important questions to consider. I discovered that it really is possible to create good arguments about right and wrong actions and to feel confidence in the resulting answers. The situations we dealt with in intensive care were tangled in the clash of perspectives that varied among caregivers, patients, and families. But philosophy provided systems of order for these perspectives. Certainly, the family's wishes, the caregiver's concerns, and the cost of this care are all important, but most important are the patient's desires. That was the answer to focus on.

My studies gave me tools that helped me organize my own thinking in addressing the ethical questions I encountered in the ICU. Consequently, I was able to help the nurses in my unit. It was all very informal at first: People who worked directly for me came to me as troubling situations occurred. But eventually, I began getting requests to assist staff in other units and to talk with members of the nonnursing staff. Hospital administrators agreed that these consultations should be organized in a way that made them available to the entire staff and to patients and families as well. Thus was the ethics consultation service created.

Because the ethics consultation service is an aspect of direct patient care, it is considered a clinical service. I share the practice with Stuart Youngner, MD, who is a psychiatrist and chair of the hospital's ethics committee, and who had been pursuing concerns similar to my own. One of us is always on call in order to make the service available around the clock. Together we field a wide range of issues, including the life-versus-death scenarios that sent me back to school. Interestingly, however, most of the questions we address involve issues of competency.

Technically, the question of a patient's competency is legal rather than ethical. It becomes ethical only when the patient makes what appears to be an unwise decision and the caregiver is uncertain whether to permit this. A classic example is a case in which the patient is a Jehovah's Witness who needs a blood transfusion. Because this religion teaches that transfusions are wrong, the patient refuses the procedure. The patient is rational, yet is making a decision that may lead to personal harm. This is a case in which both patient and caregiver require instruction. All the implications of the choice must be spelled out, but if the patient is conscious and lucid, the decision is finally his to make.

I also encounter family dilemmas that may develop when a patient has slipped into a coma and relatives are at odds over whether to continue life-sustaining technology. This is an emotionally charged situation, and the best way to begin managing it is to try to get the family to step back and look at the medical facts, the prognosis, the chances of recovery. What will the patient's quality of life be if he recovers? From there I attempt to get the family to consider what choice the patient would make — to ask whether the family's desire coincides with the patient's. This can be an uncomfortable session, but with time and careful attention to communication, it is almost always possible to resolve the conflict.

Through the ethics consultation service, I provide a considerable amount of in-service training to other hospitals in the community. We have found that the more people learn about medical ethics, the more they want to know. In fact, we just signed an agreement with a small community hospital about 40 miles from us. The hospital is too small to have its own ethics consultant, so we are going to let it tie into our service via telephone. We will visit the hospital once a month to discuss ethical issues with its staff.

While ethics takes up much of my time, it doesn't account for all my duties. In fact, while I was studying philosophy and developing the ethics consultation service I continued my ICU practice. In 1977, I assumed the role of assistant director of nursing, responsible for four (later five) ICU units. In that position, my duties were almost exclusively administrative and included fiscal management, monitoring quality of care issues, mentoring and supervising the units' head nurses, as well as overseeing policies and procedures. In that job, I began to develop an idea for a major research project.

The project responds to the shift in the types of patients seen in ICUs. Traditionally, ICU patients were critically ill, recovering from major surgeries or life-threatening conditions and physiologically very unstable. The average length of stay was about three days, after which stabilized, recovering patients would be moved to other units for less-intensive care. But more and more patients needed to stay in the ICU for weeks or even months. These patients were either recovering from surgical procedures in which there were complications, or they were older individuals with several serious problems occurring simultaneously. Ten years ago these people would have died, but now we had the knowledge and technology to not only keep them alive, but also help them recover. They needed the intensity of care provided in this type of unit, but the ICUs themselves weren't designed for long-term patients. The units are bright and noisy, people are in and out all day and night, codes and crises happen almost every hour, and family visits may be prohibited or discouraged.

Another nurse, Ellen Rudy, PhD, RN, and I recognized this problem, so we came up with the idea of creating a new environment just for these patients — a special care unit. The unit would look more like a long-term care setting, but the specialized intensive care patients needed would still be available. The unit we designed included private rooms, television sets, windows, and clocks; we encouraged a homey atmosphere — flowers, pictures of family, 24-hour visiting by family and even pets, and added facilities so family members could stay overnight. The care would be provided exclusively by nurses working in close collaboration with a medical director. In 1989 we submitted a grant proposal to the National Institutes of Health (NIH) to create a test unit of this nature. We received a $1-million grant for a three-year study of a six-patient unit. The study concludes in 1994.

The study has been fascinating. We are quantifying our cost of care, length of patient stay, complication rates, and patient satisfaction. Our preliminary findings indicate a significant reduction in costs, reduction in certain complications, especially a reduction of sepsis, and a slightly lower length of stay. The patients and families also seem more comfortable and relaxed in this atmosphere. The hospital has been enthused enough with our findings to commit space in a new wing for an eight- to 10-bed special care unit. We also published articles on our preliminary findings in *Heart and Lung* and *The Journal of Nursing Administration* — we have been inundated with requests for information from across the country. Knowing we may have created a model that will improve the care for patients throughout the country is especially exciting.

In addition to my research, administrative duties, and ethics practice, I am also an assistant professor at Case Western Reserve University's School of Nursing. I currently teach two courses on ethics, one for graduate students and one for undergraduates. I consider teaching a tremendous responsibility and a great joy. I believe the greatest influence I can have in my practice is through teaching because in teaching one student, I can eventually influence the care of many patients.

In retrospect, I probably could have chosen to be a physician or perhaps a social worker and still had a fulfilling career that centered on human care. But I don't believe either profession would have provided the opportunity or creativity I have found in nursing. I am convinced that a major reason for this lies in the preparation nurses receive as students. Medical students focus on the biological sciences, social work students concentrate on social sciences and the humanities; both are also trained in specific clinical skills. But nurses receive a balanced education that includes biological and social sciences, the humanities, and clinical skills. As a result, nurses are exceptionally well equipped to provide direct patient care and interact with patients and their families.

While the training and philosophy of nursing prepared me for such a varied career, the location of my practice has provided opportunities and let me use my own creativity. University Hospitals has a very strong nursing department, and an excellent working relationship exists among physicians, nurses, and administrators. Not many institutions in the early 1980s would have been so supportive of a nurse who decided to study philosophy in hopes of improving her clinical practice. The hospital also has a strong belief in the teaching component. In 1989, when my project was approved by NIH, I had to switch my affiliation from part-time university, full-time hospital employee to full-time university, part-time hospital employee. Again there was support from both institutions. Not all environments are so friendly to nurses. There are some empirical indicators that can tell a nurse how much nursing is valued and supported within an institution. An institution that has the chief nurse at a high level within the organization, say at the level of senior vice president, probably has more support than one that buries the chief nurse below layers of other administrators. In looking for job opportunities make sure the staff development department and its programs are well defined, respected, and supported. Discover whether there are ample support systems in place for nursing.

No matter how good the institution or how dynamic the practice, there will always be frustrations. The one I encounter most often is a lack of time. Between my ethics studies, clinical practice, teaching, and research project, it has been difficult to devote as much time to each component as I would like. For example, when I began working on my doctorate in philosophy, I had to make a 2½-hour drive twice a week to attend classes, perform my clinical duties, and teach my own course at Case Western. Currently, I maintain the ethics consultation service, am principle investigator in my research project, and teach at Case Western, all while working on my doctoral dissertation. It can be stressful, but ultimately I have found it very rewarding.

Rewards do not come without sacrifice, however, and nurses must decide early on whether their practice will be just a job, or whether it will be a career. Early in my career, the biggest "high" was saving a life, a special reward of clinical practice. But I've gone on to find other rewards, helping people with intimate personal problems, preparing students for practices of their own, and creating a new care model that may improve conditions for thousands of patients nationwide. These are the kinds of rewards that only a career can provide. And with a nursing career the opportunities are almost limitless. It really is very exciting to be right in the middle of it all.

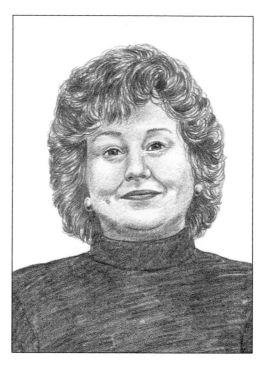

Sarah Sheets Cook, MEd, RN,C, IBCLC, FNAP,
is associate dean for academic and clinical
affairs and associate professor of
clinical nursing at Columbia University
School of Nursing in New York, New York.
She also is engaged in the
private practice of advanced
obstetrical nursing.

Obstetrics

Obstetrical nursing is basically a happy profession: Assisting a couple through a successful pregnancy and childbirth experience is truly satisfying. In addition, nursing opportunities in the obstetrics field are wide and varied, not only in terms of the type of practice but also the setting where that practice occurs.

Many obstetrical nurses practice in a hospital or birthing center setting. Here, the nurse functions as a staff member, working within the parameters of the institution's organizational structure. This may involve providing care in an antepartal or prenatal clinic, in the labor and delivery or birthing center suite, or in the newborn nursery or postpartum unit. In some institutions, staff nurses may rotate among all these units on a fixed time schedule, spending several weeks or months in each setting. In others, nurses choose the area in which they prefer to practice.

The staff nurse in an antepartal clinic assists the physician or nurse midwife in ensuring that each woman's pregnancy is progressing smoothly. Gathering information about changes since the last visit and providing counseling or answering questions are important aspects of this process. Often, women feel more comfortable talking with the nurse, because of a feeling that they might bother the physician or nurse midwife with their concerns. Skillful and compassionate nurses can not only answer questions, but can also refer questions to physicians or nurse midwives that need their input.

Working with patients at the time of birth, either in a labor and delivery unit or a birthing center suite, is always exciting; helping with the arrival of a new baby is one of life's great highs. Also, this type of practice is clinically challenging, because it is impossible to predict how a birth will progress. The nurse in labor and delivery must be prepared for anything, from assisting the physician or nurse midwife to providing support for the woman in labor.

The increasing use of technology during the birth process (eg, fetal monitoring, patient-controlled analgesia, and augmentation of slow labor) has both positive and negative aspects. In the event that the laboring woman or the baby is in difficulty, modern technology is marvelous, often making the difference between a joyous and healthy outcome and a disaster. Sometimes, however, when technology is used routinely in normal birthing situations, it can detract from the laboring woman's successful management of labor. For example, studies indicate that use of external fetal monitoring during normal situations does not produce safer or quicker births, but often slows the normal progression of labor. I can remember several instances in which I observed that nurses caring for patients in labor preferred to rely on technical equipment rather than their own assessment and evaluation skills.

One scenario I've seen more than once is that of an anxious woman in bed, connected to a fetal monitor, whose labor is not progressing. Based on my nursing assessment, I've often removed the monitor to allow the mother to get out of bed and walk around. After encouraging this ambulation and soothing her fears, I generally find that "lack of progress" swiftly changes to "ready to deliver." Nurses can make a difference.

If one likes little babies, working in the newborn nursery can be great fun. Introducing new babies to their parents and helping parents discover their child's characteristics and learn how to care for a newborn is extremely rewarding. Teaching is a large responsibility of nursery nurses who deal with topics such as how to breast feed or bathe a baby, and how the new mother can take care of herself. They also touch on the issue of how the new baby will change the family's lifestyle. Postpartum nurses usually take care exclusively of the mother who is usually exhausted and needs lots of physical care and attention. The nursery and postpartum nurses often work closely together and, in many hospitals or birthing centers, one nurse takes care of both the mother and baby.

There is another level of practice for obstetrics nurses — that of advanced clinical practice, and my own work is in this category. Sometimes this role is confused with that of a perinatal clinical nurse specialist, a neonatal clinical nurse specialist, or a nurse practitioner, all of which involve advanced education and experience in the perinatal arena. Neonatal nurse practitioners specialize in providing care for seriously ill infants in neonatal intensive care units. Their activities are similar to those of resident physicians in managing the complex technical care of such infants. But these skills are augmented by the additional caring science perspective of nurses. The role of the perinatal nurse practitioner and the clinical nurse specialist are the topics of other chapters.

My role as an advanced practice nurse in obstetrics is multifaceted. Because I am an associate professor in a major university's school of nursing, I divide my time between teaching, research, and clinical activities. I teach both basic and advanced students, focusing on content that is specific to developing, childbearing, and childrearing families. One of my courses integrates knowledge about the normal parameters of human growth and development with the science of nutrition and the promotion of health and prevention of illness. Another deals with the nutritional needs of pregnant women, and a third centers on the role of the advanced obstetrics nurse. My current research activities revolve around developing more effective ways for nurses to teach women about the importance of nutrition during pregnancy and lactation and to promote breast feeding.

Perhaps my favorite activity, and one that is integrally related to my teaching and research, is my private practice, which involves working with expectant families. I have a collaborative practice with three physicians who have a private, community-based practice in obstetrics and gynecology. I work with them in an autonomous but interdependent fashion: My clients are referred by the physicians, and I report my findings to them about patient progress and potential problems.

I provide three basic services for these families, including counseling about nutrition for pregnancy and breast feeding, preparation for childbirth education classes, and breast feeding counseling. Each woman who comes to the office for a first prenatal visit is asked to keep a record of what she eats for a week. She is also given a questionnaire that I developed to explore her feelings about and knowledge of breast feeding. After reviewing these documents, I counsel each patient and supply written materials that outline the effects of nutrition on pregnancy and breast feeding. Although some may find this nursing activity mundane, I find it challenging because each woman is different and has different educational needs, despite the similarity of all pregnancy progression.

Research indicates that the more women know about breast feeding before a baby is born, the more likely they are to be successful at breast feeding after the baby's birth. However, a number of problems can still develop. Even though both mother and baby have all the equipment needed to breast feed, they need to learn to work together in order to become an efficient breast-feeding team. That's where my counseling activities come into play. In addition to my office hours, I am available for telephone counseling, of which I do a great deal, even at the university. I also make home visits if I think it is necessary. To know that I have made a difference in helping a new mother and baby learn to work together at breast feeding is another fulfilling experience.

The childbirth education classes are small and informal, with no more than seven couples at a time. Most often, the couples are husbands and wives, but sometimes a good friend or relative will accompany a woman whose partner is unable to attend. I find it incredibly rewarding to work with couples. They arrive somewhat anxious and confused about the process of having a baby and becoming parents, but they leave feeling competent and empowered to cope with the next stage in their lives.

The classes cover information about the general progression of labor, multiple techniques for managing or coping with the process, what couples can expect in the hospital birthing center used by our practice, and what's involved in becoming parents. There are six class sessions, five of which occur before the babies are born and one that meets after the babies have arrived. In my university office, I have a large bulletin board full of pictures of my "grandchildren," those whose parents attended my classes. By now, I am a grandma of some 400 kids.

Many educational paths lead to obstetrics nursing. Basic nursing programs (diploma, associate degree, and baccalaureate — to which I am partial) all provide enough education about obstetrics to enable graduates to function as staff nurses. Advanced education, either master's or doctoral studies, is necessary for nurses who wish to pursue an advanced role. Specialty board certification, similar to physicians' specialty certification, is also available and useful for nurses in advanced practice.

For those who wonder if I have a life of my own, the answer is that of course I do. I'm a wife and mother as well as an advanced clinical specialist in obstetrics nursing. The profession of nursing provides incredible variety and fulfillment in a way that no other profession, including medicine, does.

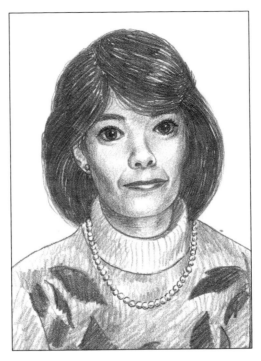

Mary Byrne, PhD, RN,
is director of the Entry to Practice and
the Master's Perinatal Programs at
Columbia University School of Nursing,
New York, New York.

Pediatrics

Good pediatrics nurses never forget two important facts about their patients. The first is that children are not miniature adults. The second is that patients in a pediatric unit should be viewed as children who happen to be sick. Simplistic as these axioms may sound, they suggest that beyond having an understanding of pediatric disease, practitioners in this area must be expert in child development — and they must use considerable finesse in applying that expertise.

Illness can have more profound psychological impact on children than on adults. Indeed, chronic disease is likely to impair a child's physical and emotional development to some degree. Consequently, a significant challenge for pediatrics nurses in a hospital is to create as much normalcy as possible in a forbidding environment that is not necessarily conducive to normal development. Insofar as it can be, the pediatric ward should be a place of happiness and activity in order to mitigate the negative effect it can have on a sick child.

The concept of an interdisciplinary approach to patient care is much in vogue. But in pediatrics this can make the difference between adequate and exceptional care. The sharp assessment skills a pediatrics nurse needs depend on refined knowledge about physiology, pharmacology, and pediatric growth and development. But equally important is a strong understanding of psychology, sociology, and anthropology — all of which enable the nurse to appreciate the significance of certain behaviors, family values, and cultural differences.

Clinically, there are significant differences between children and adults, and the margin for error can be extremely narrow in the pediatric patient. For instance, the fact that a child's body has a relatively small mass in comparison with its skin surface can have a great impact on the principles of fluid balances. As a result, only a few cubic centimeters of fluid — an amount that might be insignificant in an adult — can be vital for a pediatric patient. That's why diarrhea that would be relatively nonthreatening in an adult can be fatal in a child. That also is why the pediatrics nurse should double check all medication doses, regardless of who calculated them.

One of the myths in pediatric nursing is that experience in an adult medical-surgical unit is prerequisite. I believe the reverse can be true: The clinical precision one acquires while addressing the rapid physiologic changes that occur with pediatric growth is a superb asset for nurses who care for adult patients.

Safety is a large issue in a pediatric unit, and ensuring it often means controlling the activities of patients. Babies need crib rails; older children have to be discouraged from running in the halls. Children's behavior also may place them at greater risk for infection than adults. Moreover, they lack judgement abilities. For instance, a nurse might instruct a child not to eat. But it would be naive to believe the child will remember or obey every instruction, so supervision is required.

Pediatric patients often have difficulty expressing themselves effectively. They may be reluctant to admit they're afraid. They may not be able to communicate the fact that they are in pain. In fact, they may not even realize they are in pain, particularly if they have suffered with a chronically painful disease. Because of this, pain monitoring has become an important issue in pediatrics. For years, pain was overlooked in pediatric patients, partly because the psychology of children was not well understood, and partly because adults didn't want to believe they were contributing to a child's pain. In acute care areas, including pediatric intensive care units, the focus on survival is so sharp that pain sometimes is regarded as a necessary price to pay. That attitude may be appropriate with an adult patient who understands the concept of long-term consequences. But children find it far more difficult to temper their immediate experience with thoughts of the future. Even so, children seemingly have a remarkable ability to deal well with terrible things. When painful procedures are necessary, every effort should be made to perform them in places other than the child's room; the child's room and bed always should represent safety and comfort. And just as hospitalized children need special safe places, so do pediatrics nurses — places away from the bedside where they can vent their emotions.

Empathy is essential in any nursing field, but nowhere is it more important than in pediatric nursing. Because many of their patients cannot communicate verbally, pediatrics nurses must have an innate or an acquired understanding of what their patients are experiencing.

Most of the nurse's time is spent directly with children in the pediatric unit. Some of this time is devoted to such specific nursing tasks as administering tests or treatments, but much of it is simply spending time with the child to provide comfort, explanations, or stimulation. A nurse might play peek-a-boo with an infant while checking his isolation precautions, or use a game to explain diabetic diet management to a group of school-age children. During a busy period, a fretful toddler may be planted in his stroller in the middle of the nurses' station, where he can be watched closely. Change-of-shift reports usually take the form of walking rounds that let young patients see who will be taking care of them. These rounds also give the nurse an opportunity to see and assess each child.

Physicians often rely heavily on pediatrics nurses. In fact, some physicians won't touch a child unless the nurse is present because they know the nurse has established a strong bond of trust with the child. As important as it is for nurses to bond with patients, it's also important to know other children in the unit well enough to interpret a patient's behavior in terms of the group. Children connect with one another without the ritual and social rules adults require. They talk to each other and interact much more freely than adults. Indeed, they often create an entire culture on a unit that the nurse may or may not be aware of. As a result, the best pediatrics nurses become attuned to group dynamics and are able to balance the needs of the individual against the needs of the unit. A good pediatrics nurse will spend time planning activities and working with outside specialists, including teachers, to implement activities on the unit. In addition, establishing rules and defining good behavior are part of the pediatrics nurse's job.

Nowhere is patience a greater virtue than in pediatrics nursing — not the teeth-clenching, grin-and-bear-it kind, but a patience that recognizes children as growing persons who are not yet adults. Such patience includes an optimism for what all children can become. Uncompromising honesty is another vital quality, because children are usually open with people and expect the same in return. The pediatrics nurse must never lie to children about what they will experience, because honesty is the foundation for the trusting relationship required to promote healing. Breaches of this trust are virtually impossible to repair.

Pediatrics nursing is actually a misnomer that defines the specialty in medical language, implying an acute inpatient care setting. In fact, we prefer the term *child health specialist,* which suggests an overall concern with health that crosses settings and results in a continuum of care. Issues involving children's health cannot be limited to the boundaries of the pediatric ward, but must cross over into the realms of family planning, pregnancy, birth, growth, and development. Also, not only must the pathology and the medical diagnosis of injury or illness be considered, so must the patient's and the family's responses to it.

A pediatrics nurse must elicit information from parents and include them from the beginning of a child's care. In the admission interview, the nurse might ask parents about rituals at home — such as a bedtime story — or whether the child has a nickname. Hospitalized children need to feel connected to their normal family environments, and parents need to feel part of the hospital routine.

It usually is wise to talk with parents and children separately as well as together in order that they may talk candidly about their concerns and fears. Especially with adolescents, it may be well to interview the child privately, remembering that there is a fine line between respecting the privacy of each patient and ignoring the parent-child relationship. Feelings of jealousy are not uncommon in parents who feel the nurse is usurping their natural role. The nurse must be alert for this attitude and skillfully include the parent if it appears to be developing.

A pediatrics nurse's involvement will vary according to the length of a patient's stay in the hospital. With a brief stay, the nurse must initiate teaching plans and make referrals so that other providers — other nurses or family members — can be entrusted with continued care. With longer or recurring hospitalizations, the nurse who gets to know the family more intimately will be able to make more comprehensive assessments.

Inpatient settings, of course, are not the only practice choice for pediatrics nurses. They may work in outpatient clinics, in schools, in physicians' offices, or in home care. There's a growing need for pediatrics nurses to provide health education in schools and other community settings. Some advanced practice pediatrics nurses even combine activities from a variety of settings.

The pediatrics nurse who practices in an outpatient setting needs a clinical background that is no less strong than the inpatient nurse's. In fact, in an isolated primary care setting, where it may be difficult to get backup and second opinions, the nurse may find this foundation even more important.

Professional disillusionment in any specialty is a function of a nurse's original expectations. For example, the pediatrics nurse should expect to provide care for children with all kinds of problems, but it would be unrealistic to imagine all can be cured. Pain, discomfort, and death are among life's harsh realities, and a pediatrics nurse will encounter all of them. To experience a child's suffering is heartbreaking, but nurses must learn to provide a caring presence, even when cure is not possible.

The most pressing concerns in contemporary health care are those of access and resource allocation within an environment of cost containment. And, pediatric care will not escape the scrutiny this produces. Consequently, it is incumbent on pediatrics nurses to seek a voice in defining what is necessary to ensure the health of our children. In doing so, they will exert a large influence on our society's most precious resource. As tomorrow's health care system evolves, pediatrics nurses — especially those in advanced practice — will have an important role to play in caring for this population. The career opportunities that result will be full of challenge and excitement.

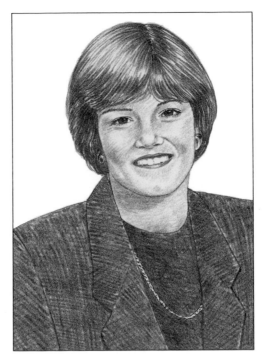

*Terry T. Fulmer, PhD, RN, FAAN,
is the Anna C. Maxwell Professor of
Nursing Research, and associate dean
for research at Columbia University
School of Nursing, New York, New York.*

Geriatrics

The mission of gerontological nursing is to improve the quality of life and quality of care for patients over the age of 65. Because geriatric care is population specific, nurses have almost unlimited opportunities for careers that are challenging and rewarding. They can practice with great autonomy, work as members of multidisciplinary teams, or participate in traditional care structures. From clinical care and specialized research to education and administration, the practice options available to geriatrics nurses are vast. And so is the array of practice settings: home care, day care, hospitals, long-term care facilities, and outpatient clinics. There is a gerontological practice to suit almost any professional interest. The demand for nurses in this field is strong, and because the population of geriatric Americans will nearly double in the next 30 years, it will increase steadily.

Age does not equal disease, nor does normal aging encompass disease. In the past, medical professionals made the mistake of believing certain diseases (anemia, for example) were natural by-products of the aging process. Indeed, there is great heterogeneity in the way people age. There are extremely vigorous 80-year-olds and very debilitated 65-year-olds. Much of a good geriatrics nurse's skill lies in assessing the patient's presentations and determining which are attributable to aging and which to disease.

This is not always an easy task. Elderly adults may suffer from strokes, fractures and other acute conditions, or temporary mobility problems, and these often will be exacerbated by a mix of chronic problems that include arthritis, memory loss, heart disease, and declining vision and hearing. In addition, those who care for the elderly have to contend with the fact that diseases may present differently in a geriatric patient than in a younger adult. For instance, the older patient with pneumonia may be afebrile and may present with no cough, only slight congestion, and, perhaps, a confused mental state.

The geriatric patient also responds differently to drug therapy. Dosages that would be well within acceptable levels for a young adult may be too large for the aged person. For these reasons, those who provide care for the elderly require specialized training and significant experience with this population.

Because of their expertise in functional assessment, nurses are especially well suited to caring for the elderly. From initial estimation of functionality, to evaluation of a patient's recovery from acute events, to the continuing appraisal of daily living skills, assessment is at the heart of this specialty.

I also believe that nursing education produces an advantageous foundation for gerontological practice. While physician training generally concentrates on treatment of disease states and subspecialty activities, the nurse is taught to provide the comprehensive care these patients need. Nurses are schooled in health practice and disease prevention along with the basic pathology of disease states.

A baccalaureate program provides the basic gerontological education nurses need; clinical experience gained by working with elderly patients will sharpen their assessment skills and other abilities. But for nurses who want to specialize in gerontological nursing, certification and graduate preparation for advanced practice are recommended.

The American Nurses Association offers three levels of certification in gerontological nursing: gerontological nurse, geriatrics nurse practitioner (GNP), and gerontological clinical nurse specialist (GNS). Certification as a gerontological nurse is based on a comprehensive examination. Certification as a GNP or GNS requires postgraduate study. Some schools of nursing urge interested undergraduate students to begin working toward this certification directly after graduation from a baccalaureate program. In an effort to enhance credentialing of their staffs, some nursing homes and hospitals provide classes for nurses who wish to become certified. In addition, many continuing education programs provide instruction in gerontological nursing.

All GNP and GNS programs are designed to help nurses acquire specialized skills in physical, functional, and psychosocial assessment of elderly patients. In addition, these programs offer advanced instruction in pathophysiology and pharmacology as they relate to older adults. Behavioral concerns also receive strong emphasis. All programs require clinical rotations.

On average, both graduate and certificate education take one year to complete. In 1990, nurses who wanted to become GNPs could choose among 28 academic programs. Approximately 40 percent of graduates found employment at nursing homes or with physicians working in nursing homes. Some 35 percent accepted positions in inner-city facilities including hospitals and clinics, while 20 percent chose rural areas for their practices. As of this writing, over 30 states currently have granted prescriptive authority to NPs.

Currently, nearly 42 percent of acute care patients who are admitted to hospitals are 65 and over. These patients tend to have more complex illnesses than younger patients. In fact, the average length of stay for elderly patients is 8.9 days — for younger adults, it's 5.6 days.

Almost 45 percent of all ICU patients are elderly.

Many hospitals employ geriatrics clinical nurses. Increasingly, such specialists are unit based and provide a combination of direct and indirect care. On geriatric units, medical and orthopedic units, and in ICUs, elderly patients may present with conditions so complicated that the hospital uses master's-level gerontological nurses as case managers. These nurses work with primary nurses and directly with older patients in order to ensure key gerontological concepts are employed.

In nursing homes, the skills of advanced practice GNPs are especially sought. At any given time, 1.5 million patients (some seven percent of our entire elderly population) are being cared for in U.S. nursing homes. Most of these patients are very sick and frail, and the complexity of their cases makes for a challenging practice.

Caring for the very ill is only one aspect of a nursing home practice. Many people in these facilities are there for short-term convalescence. Hospitalization would be inappropriate for these recovering patients, but they still need specialized care. The nurse plays an essential part in their rehabilitation by assessing their progress, helping them regain the ability to perform activities of daily life, and working with outside resources to facilitate a safe and comfortable return home.

Given the heavy regulation, reimbursement structure and the fear the public generally has of nursing homes, much is needed in the way of health policy for long-term care and public education. It is remarkable what long-term care nurses accomplish. One of their challenges today is to maintain patients in nursing homes during the final days of their lives instead of sending them to hospitals to die, which has been a practice in the past.

GNPs and GNSs provide services in a variety of settings, including public and private clinics, VA facilities, and private physicians' offices. In these locations, GNSs maintain their own case loads and collaborate with physicians. At many sites — rural and urban — the GNP or GNS may offer the only access to care for elderly adults. Additional opportunities are becoming available in over 12,000 home care agencies throughout the country.

Many nontraditional practice opportunities are also opening up for the geronotological nurse. Foremost among these are continuing care retirement communities, which form a bridge between independent living and placement in a nursing home. People in these communities are no longer able to live at home alone, but they still are active and healthy enough to be relatively independent within a framework of specialized services. In continuing care communities, GNPs and GNSs are recognized as effective providers of high-quality, cost-effective services. They perform similar roles in many adult day care centers.

Growing numbers of geriatrics nurse practitioners are developing ambulatory practices and consultancies to augment existing community services. For instance, GNPs may forge relationships with clinics or physicians in which nurses provide assessment and treatment services for patients with such age-related conditions as urinary incontinence or dementia. Under health care reform, this is likely to become a predominant model.

There are additional opportunities in research. In fact, the National Institute on Aging currently has a research grant budget of approximately $400 million. Of the many topics under investigation, preventing abuse of the elderly is one in which nurses have had substantial impact. Gerontological nurses also have made significant contributions to research on Alzheimer's disease, elder abuse, the use of restraints, and other issues related to the care of the elderly.

The elderly in our society have traditionally been undervalued as people and victims of ageism. Gerontological nurses will continue to be influential in bringing about change and a more positive focus on geriatric health issues.

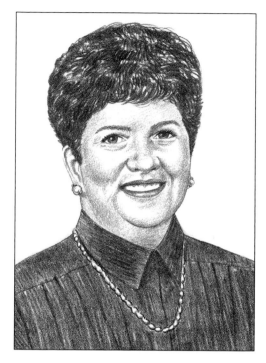

Sheila Sparks, DNSc, RN, CS,
is an assistant professor at
Georgetown University School of Nursing in
Washington, D.C.

Rehabilitation

Measuring not in yards or feet, but in inches—that's what rehabilitation nursing is all about. Taking tiny steps forward, such as picking up a fork or sitting up in bed, may not mean much to most people, but for rehabilitation nurses enormous fulfillment lies in these small accomplishments. In the short run, rehabilitation nursing may lack the drama of the intensive care unit or the emergency room, but in the long run, the rewards of this specialty are difficult to find elsewhere.

Rehabilitation nurses work to preserve patients' function, minimize further loss of ability, and promote independence. They work as case managers, caregivers, teachers, counselors, consultants, and researchers, relying on a variety of skills that are easily transferred to other areas of nursing. No matter what my job—from head nurse of a rehabilitation unit to my current position as an assistant professor teaching medical-surgical nursing at Georgetown University's School of Nursing—I've been able to apply the principles of rehabilitation nursing.

I completed a diploma program of nursing in 1968, graduated with a BSN in 1977, an MSN in 1980, and a doctorate of nursing science in 1990. I'm also certified as a medical-surgical clinical nurse specialist. I received my introduction to rehabilitation nursing when I was asked to head a brand-new rehabilitation unit. There, working primarily with individuals who had had strokes, spinal cord injuries (SCI), or head injuries, I found myself in an area of nursing that had a profound effect on whether or not clients would adapt successfully to life following their injury or illness.

The rehabilitation nurse must be willing and able to deal with the whole person. In this field, you will have extended contact with patients, working with them for weeks or months at a time. As a result, it's important that you get to know patients on their own terms. For example, I remember a quadriplegic patient who was very angry and depressed about his injury, and was verbally abusive to the nurse who cared for him. She found it difficult to deal with him day after day, but she persevered. Eventually, he began to be more cooperative and started making progress in his rehabilitation. When I asked why his behavior changed so markedly, he told me that the nurse's attitude had a lot to do with it. "No matter what I dished out," he said, "she kept coming back. She refused to give up, and she helped me see that I was a worthwhile person."

Rehabilitation nurses must try diligently to understand their patients' behavior and to pick up on the cues they give. Once, I had two young males with spinal cord injuries who went down to the hospital snack room. When they came back, they were clearly angry and went straight to bed, refusing to talk to anyone. It turned out that the person at the counter had treated them as second-class citizens. I said that, unfortunately, they probably would encounter this behavior from time to time, and we discussed ways of responding to it. Then, as the head nurse and part of the hospital's administrative team, I talked about the incident with the other department heads and suggested we should provide in-service training to teach their staff how to treat people in wheelchairs.

As staff nurses are oriented into rehabilitation, they gradually begin to spend time working with the interdisciplinary team and understanding the contributions of each member. That's a basic concept in rehabilitation nursing: No single person can do it alone. After six or nine months, the rehabilitation nurse should have acquired a good sense of how to develop realistic goals for clients. The aim is to progress from short-term, interim goals toward a long-term one, remembering that all are markers in themselves.

A rehabilitation clinical nurse specialist works closely with other hospital personnel in providing care. For instance, when a person with a stroke is admitted, it is necessary to work with nurses from ICU, emergency, medical-surgical and other departments to develop a plan for care and to make sure the patient is scheduled for physical, occupational, and speech therapy as early as possible.

A rehabilitation nurse also works with families, instructing them in necessary details about patients' conditions and problems they might encounter. Many families find it difficult to allow an SCI or stroke patient to become independent, but the nurse teaches them that often the best action is inaction — letting patients do for themselves, even if it takes longer. Children especially need to understand this. Otherwise, they might think their mother is being mean by not helping their father put on his shirt when he is capable of doing so. In counseling sessions, the rehabilitation nurse makes sure the entire family understands the goal of rehabilitation.

The skills of a detective are useful in this field, because it is important to know whether the family is continuing to care properly for the patient after discharge. For instance, some patients are embarrassed to have their families do bowel care, and if the family doesn't carry it out, the consequences can be serious. The rehabilitation nurse must be aware of such circumstances and find a solution by working through the problem with the patient and family, or by finding an alternate care provider — a home care nurse, for example. If family members think it doesn't matter whether routines are occasionally interrupted, they don't understand the seriousness of the consequences. It's the nurse's job to make sure they do.

A clinical nurse specialist probably will be involved in support groups for patients and their families. For instance, wives of male patients might meet with a nurse to discuss their concerns about sexual relations, the progress of their husband's recovery, and even such matters as managing the household finances if that is a task the husband used to do. Often, they want to find a way to make their husbands feel they're still contributing to the family.

The best rehabilitation nurses are characterized by their patients, because in this practice it is important to take it slow—to give the patient time to do everything possible for himself. Otherwise, we may condition people to be unnecessarily dependent. If it takes a patient an hour to get dressed by himself, give him the hour. Stepping in to help get the day started faster does not expedite the rehabilitation process. The nurse should always be questioning whether the patient could feed himself if given enough time; whether he could take a shower alone if he used a chair; whether he really needs to be in bed. Because patients in rehabilitation are suffering from massive loss of independence, a good nurse will find ways to involve them in their recovery whenever possible.

By the same token, hospital schedules should not be imposed on a patient; the patient's personal routines should take precedence. For instance, if a patient is accustomed to performing bowel care at night, the nurse shouldn't insist that it be done in the morning. It's likely that the patient has a good reason for his schedule, and disrupting his routine will only make it harder to reestablish it at home.

Rehabilitation nurses work in inpatient acute care hospitals, freestanding rehabilitation facilities, and nursing homes. While the basic skills required are the same in every setting, a nurse who works with hospitalized patients is more engaged in direct care and education. An outpatient nurse probably focuses more on evaluating the patient's progress, determining compliance with discharge instructions, and detecting complications. In a nursing home, the nurse will be involved with problems that are common in elderly populations. Because so many incapacitating injuries are accident induced, prevention is an important area of rehabilitation, and many nurses give safety seminars at schools in their communities.

A full range of nursing skills is exercised in rehabilitation. Psychological support is a huge component, especially with stroke or head injury patients whose cognitive functions have been impaired. And, because patients may be affected by other medical conditions as well, the nurse in this specialty needs a good foundation in medical-surgical nursing. A creative spirit also helps encourage patients to continue striving for difficult goals. Just as important is the ability to be a team player, sharing successes and recognizing the contributions of others.

The slowness with which progress is made is easily the most frustrating aspect of rehabilitation nursing. But this is more than offset by the tremendous satisfaction that comes with knowing I've helped a patient get better. I remember one patient who had made wonderful progress: She was walking, putting on her clothes, and learning to use eating utensils. Still, she was depressed. I talked with her and discovered that those achievements meant little to her because what she really wanted was a far different triumph: She wanted to smile for her husband.

After I learned this, I worked with her every night, helping her put on lipstick and practice smiling in a mirror. Within several weeks, she was able to manage a smile — and it meant more to her than being able to walk. As I said, success in this work is measured in inches.

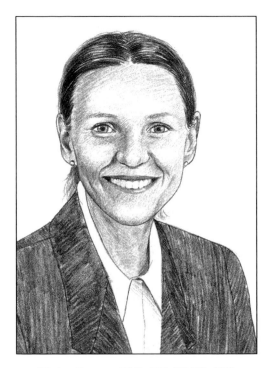

Elaine Larson, PhD, RN, FAAN, CIC,
is dean and professor at the
Georgetown University School of Nursing,
Washington, D.C.

Infection Control

Nurses' earliest responsibilities were to give comfort, provide cleansing and physical care, and prevent complications, particularly infections, among those patients in their charge. While the prevention of infection and the control of its spread has traditionally been a responsibility of all professional nurses, during the 1960s this increasingly complex task developed into a specialty practice. In 1993, there were approximately 10,000 practitioners of infection control; more than 90 percent are registered nurses.

Late in the 1950s, one of the first textbooks on nosocomial infections was published. During that time and into the 1960s, the high cost — in dollars and in health — of these infections became clear, primarily as a result of pandemics of staphylococcal infections in newborn nurseries and operating rooms. At the time, large tertiary care centers began to designate one individual, a physician or nurse, to monitor infections and to implement policies and procedures that could reduce rates of infection. Then in the late 1960s, the Joint Commission on Accreditation of Hospitals required every hospital to have an infection control committee and to implement infection prevention and control policies. This mandate created a need for an expanded pool of professionals with specific skills in epidemiology, microbiology, and infection control.

In 1970, the Centers for Disease Control (CDC) began the National Nosocomial Infection Surveillance study and initiated efforts to standardize surveillance and control activities. As part of this effort, CDC offered courses in epidemiology to train infection control practitioners (ICPs). By mid-decade, virtually every medium-to-large hospital had at least one of these specialists on staff. Nurses were recognized as the most appropriate health professionals to assume leadership in this specialty because of their intimate knowledge of patient care and their familiarity with hospital systems. A landmark study conducted by the CDC and published in 1981, the *Study of Efficacy of Nosocomial Infection Control* (SENIC), demonstrated a significant reduction in nosocomial infection rates in hospitals that had certain characteristics, one of which was the presence of an ICP for every 250 beds. With this study, the role of the ICP in the reduction of nosocomial infection rates and costs associated with these infections was unequivocally demonstrated, and the specialty was firmly established.

The role of the ICP has been evolving ever since. Initially, this clinical practice focused on the investigation of infectious outbreaks in hospitals; surveillance of all hospitalized patients in an effort to identify all infections; microbiologic monitoring of the hospital environment (sinks, floors, and equipment); and routine microbiologic culturing of selected high-risk populations (eg, newborns). In the 1980s, more targeted methods of surveillance, such as identifying only selected marker infections, and surveillance by objective, moved the specialty away from ritualistic and cost-intensive and labor-intensive methods to a more thoughtful and outcome-oriented approach. Even now, standards of practice are being developed by the CDC and by the Association for Practitioners in Infection Control and Epidemiology, and are being validated with clinical studies. In addition to surveillance of infection, ICPs spend a major portion of their time educating health care personnel in policies, procedures, and practices that minimize the risk of infection.

In recent years, the specialty of infection control has been influenced by two major events: the HIV epidemic and the change in financing of health care. The increase in AIDS cases has drawn attention to the importance of infection control practices and standards and to the central contributions of infection control nurses as leaders, teachers, and monitors in this area. The focus on HIV also has drawn significant attention to the protection of the health care professional as well as the patient, and a plethora of new concerns, guidelines, and regulations are being interpreted and managed by the ICP.

Changes in health care financing and the current effort to cut costs have had substantial impact on the scope of the ICP's practice. To their duties in surveillance and outcomes measurement, these nurses have added responsibilities in financial management, and more generally, in quality assessment.

The *American Journal of Infection Control* and *Infection Control and Hospital Epidemiology* publish a variety of articles about this specialty. The contents of these national journals attest to the broad scope of current practice of the ICP, which frequently includes research as well as data gathering for continued monitoring.

There are no specific educational requirements for the nurse who is interested in the specialty of infection control. This is an interdisciplinary field, including primarily registered nurses, but also medical technologists, microbiologists, and infectious disease physicians. Most infection control nurses hold at least a baccalaureate in nursing, although this is not mandatory. Several schools of nursing offer specialty training at the master's-degree level; other nurses seek master's preparation in public health or epidemiology to enhance their quantitative skills and professional status. Many ICPs receive their initial training on the job, then go on for formal training through continuing education courses, advanced education, or certification.

The need for ICPs is increasing and will remain high as efforts intensify to contain costs. This practice offers nurses exceptional independence, unusual visibility, and an opportunity to create measurable change in the health care environment.

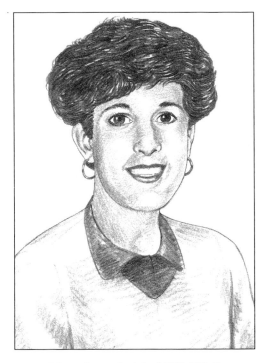

Mary Agnes Ostick, MSN, RN,C,
is an adult nurse practitioner for
CamCare Corporation in
Camden, New Jersey.

Adult Nurse Practitioner

I have enjoyed every nursing job I've ever had, but my last 10 years as a nurse practitioner have been particularly rewarding. The basic science component that underlies nursing has always held my interest, and my role as a nurse practitioner draws on this knowledge every day. In order to remain current in my field, I am constantly learning. And I'm in a clinical setting where I can see at first hand the value of my efforts. When I began my nursing career, nurse practitioners were not commonplace. It was not until several years later that their importance was widely recognized.

I completed a diploma program in 1974, worked in an emergency room, and then moved to a coronary care unit. There, I worked with a director who believed nurses should be utilized to their full potential. He thought that because nurses often were at the bedside when problems occurred, they were in an ideal position to save patients' lives. During my six-year tenure in the CCU, I learned to appreciate how much impact a nurse's skills could have in life-threatening situations.

Consequently, I decided to go back to school for my BSN and took a full-time job as a school nurse. I was surprised to discover that I enjoyed working outside the hospital, and I realized that a nurse's activities don't always have to be performed at the bedside. I could consult with a pediatrician over the phone when necessary, but I was the school's sole health care provider. In addition to assessing students' acute illnesses, I spent a large amount of time teaching formally in the classroom and informally in my office. I didn't know it at the time, but I was performing some functions that are similar to those of a nurse practitioner.

In 1982, I received my BSN and accepted a teaching position in critical care nursing at the diploma school I had attended. As much as I enjoyed working with students and sharing my knowledge, I soon began to miss providing patient care.

I knew that if I wanted to continue to advance professionally, I would need a master's degree. I borrowed some money and enrolled in the graduate program at the University of Pennsylvania. I intended to become a cardiovascular clinical nurse specialist, which was a natural extension of my background in coronary care. Nevertheless, early in the program, I began to want a completely new challenge, and the nurse practitioner program caught my eye. It placed a strong emphasis on basic pathology and science, and the concept of learning physical assessment skills was exciting. I figured that what I could learn in this program would be valuable if I returned to teaching. So I took the plunge and transferred to the primary care adult nurse practitioner program.

At the time, nurse practitioners were just beginning to surface in the medical community. I felt that nurses who entered this pioneer profession would have to do a fair amount of trailblazing before achieving general acceptance. I wasn't sure that I wanted to be part of this movement, but I liked what they were learning and doing.

The physician who precepted me at CamCare taught me a great deal and had a significant impact on my career. He supported the nurse practitioner program and saw nurse practitioners as a way to help the underserved populations of the inner city. He also believed in me, always urging me to read more and to refine my skills. I grew to love the scientific challenge as well as the daily contact with patients.

Ten years later I'm still here, although both the center and my work in it have changed. When I first came to CamCare, we operated a small clinic out of an old church. Since then, the center has relocated to a new building and has expanded to several other sites.

The health center serves a diverse urban population that, in general, is not oriented to healthy lifestyles and practices. People usually don't visit the clinic for a yearly physical; they come in when they're sick. As is the case in any urban setting, there has been an increase in drug abuse and associated health problems. AIDS, hepatitis, and other comunicable diseases remain a threat. Immunization for children has to be a priority in order to prevent childhood diseases such as measles.

When I first started working here, I often found myself emotionally overwhelmed by the adversity our patients must deal with. Over the years, I've worked to become a part of these people's lives. I've watched their kids grow up, and they have given me baby showers. At Christmas, they bake cookies for me. As frustrating as it is not to be able to change the social problems that are directly or indirectly responsible for many of the health problems I see, I love my job.

I work 24 hours a week, seeing 12 to 16 patients each day, many of whom are walk-ins. We have seven physicians and four nurse practitioners as well as a nurse manager and technicians. As a primary care provider, I perform many of the same tasks physicians do. The scope of my practice encompasses acute illness as well as chronic stable illness. When patients require more complex management, I involve a physician, either by referring the patient or requesting a consultation. When I came here in 1984, I worried that the other health care providers might not accept me, but I found just the opposite to be true.

During visits, I take a medical history and interview patients about their lifestyles, including diet, exercise, and sleep habits. Then I perform a physical exam that may include heart-lung auscultation and a funduscopic exam. I look for signs of organ damage that is secondary to diabetes and hypertension, because these conditions are prevalent in my patients. I may order additional lab tests, EKGs, or x-rays before making my assessment.

Consulting among the health care professionals in our clinic is an integral part of our practice. I consult not only with the doctors, but with the other nurse practitioners, and sometimes the doctors seek out our advice and expertise. For example, the physicians often refer their women patients to us for routine gynecology care or their women's health issues.

In general, nurse practitioners have responsibility for patient education, because it has been a traditional component of nursing education. In our office, for example, the goal with newly diagnosed diabetic patients is to keep them independent by teaching them to recognize symptoms that indicate problems, how to administer insulin, and when to call the provider.

A significant part of my job is serving as a gatekeeper and guide through the health care maze. In that way, I become patients' advocate. I am their link to other health care providers and social service agencies.

Nurse practitioners fill a growing need in primary care. Because of our cost effectiveness, we are especially valuable in underserved areas. And as physicians continue the trend toward specialization, the need for general primary care providers is growing. Nurse practitioners are filling that need. We are not physicians — we are nurses who have moved up another rung on the career ladder. We have more autonomy and more education, and we have become more medically competent while retaining our nursing foundation.

Nurse practitioners can work in a variety of settings. In addition to primary care facilities, they often work in schools, where they perform annual physicals, take care of students' basic health needs, and provide education about prevention. Industry is another growing area of opportunity, and nurse practitioners in occupational health settings work for companies, conducting physicals, managing routine care, and implementing preventive care programs. Also, because emergency rooms are glutted with primary care cases, some hospitals have established fast-track emergency rooms staffed with nurse practitioners. In addition, nurse practitioners can concentrate on a number of clinical areas, including women's health, family health, geriatrics, and pediatrics.

Reimbursement for services is a critical issue for nurse practitioners. Currently, my earnings come from my practice, not from third-party payers. Reimbursement for nurse practitioners differs from state to state. The resolution of this dilemma will have a far-reaching impact on the profession. In the meantime, I can tell that we are no longer pioneers, but have gained professional status and acceptance. I used to have to explain what I do for a living . . . but not any more.

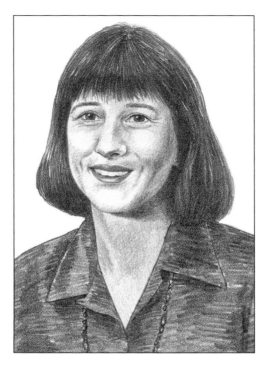

Margaret E. Rogers, MS, RN, CFNP,
practices at Montefiore Family Health Center
in the Bronx, New York, and
is an instructor in clinical nursing at
Columbia University School of Nursing,
New York, New York.

Family Nurse Practitioner

When I became interested in nursing, I wanted to find a challenging career in which I could actively help people and serve the community. I also wanted a profession that would give me a great deal of self-determination, both in my daily practice activities and in my choice of practice site. I wasn't sure that a single practice could meet these requirements, but as a family nurse practitioner I've found a perfect fit. My patients, most of whom are poor, have been an even greater reward. They inspire me. As I've watched them struggle against tremendous odds, they've never failed to display great dignity and pride.

A family nurse practitioner (FNP) is engaged in an advanced practice that focuses on cradle-to-grave primary care. This nurse diagnoses and treats patients holistically, considering not only the symptoms and disease, but the influence of family relations, social pressures, and work environments. A typical practice involves both acute and chronic conditions, but there is generally a strong emphasis on prevention.

I embarked on my own career more than 12 years ago. Several years after majoring in Spanish literature as an undergraduate, I was attracted to an unusual nursing program. A BSN was not required for entry, and two and a half years of intensive clinical and academic studies would produce a master's degree as well as FNP certification. As I began my studies, I discovered that, unlike hospital settings, where patients tend to be very sick and unempowered, patients in a family nurse practitioner's practice are mostly healthy. Even better, the practitioners use their skills to make sure the patients stay healthy. The more I learned about it, the more certain I was that this was the career for me.

Today, my practice is at the Montefiore Family Health Center in the Bronx, New York. The center is an ambulatory care clinic, and our patients come from the surrounding neighborhoods, which are poor and represent different racial and ethnic goups. Most of our patients rely on Medicaid or belong to a Bronx-based HMO/Medicaid program. For those who don't have access to any type of third-party reimbursement, we charge on a sliding scale based on their ability to pay. Most of our patients are children and young women, but we provide care for family members of all ages.

By and large, people in the socioeconomic group we care for avoid seeking medical care until they absolutely need it. However, our adult patients have become pretty good about scheduling annual checkups for themselves and periodic visits for their children. At least in part, we attribute this to the strong bonds of trust we've been able to establish with patients. They see the same caregiver every time they come in, so they feel comfortable with us. We try to build on these relationships and instill a belief in the need for regular medical care.

About four years ago we exceeded our capacity and had to stop accepting new patients. Now, we accept new members only from families we already serve, and for special projects being run by the HMO or Montefiore. As a result, our patients have established relationships with practitioners here.

The center is a multidisciplinary practice with a family nurse practitioner, family practice physicians, a psychologist, social workers, and medical assistants all working together. I have my own case load and I take histories, make diagnoses, and develop plans for patient care. Because I am fluent in Spanish, I treat many of our Hispanic patients.

Appointment hours are Monday through Friday, between 9 AM and 5 PM. I see patients after one of our medical assistants has acquired baseline information (determined their weight, blood pressure, temperature) and completed documentation.

Most of my visits involve reviewing the patient's chief complaint, taking a history, performing a physical exam, rendering a diagnosis, and recommending therapies or treatments. Nothing, however, is quite this simple or straightforward. Patient encounters are always challenging, in part because of the diverse patient population we serve. I see everything from colds and routine new-job physicals to patients who have been recently diagnosed as HIV positive. This is unlike many nursing specialties that focus on one particular gender, age group, or disease state.

Another challenge lies in the philosophy associated with this type of practice. Because we diagnose and treat the whole patient, rather than just the symptoms, external factors in patients' lives, including family dynamics, current living environment, and other outside stressors, are important. As a result, the practitioner needs to quickly establish a rapport with patients and try to uncover hidden reasons contributing to their visit.

One of the highlights of my practice is doing prenatal care. Once pregnancy is verified, women visit once a month during the first seven months, every other week during month eight, and then every week for the last month. These visits include monitoring weight, blood pressure, and lab values to detect such diseases as gestational diabetes. We monitor fetal growth and I check for indications of fetal health. During each visit, I educate patients about the importance of proper nutrition and general health care for both mother and child. At the same time, I offer strong cautions against smoking, alcohol, and drug abuse. We encourage all pregnant women to participate in the center's childbirth preparation classes.

Women with high-risk pregnancies require more frequent monitoring. I take similar precautions with pregnant adolescents, especially those who are having their first child. Because these young women are likely to need help with emotional issues, financial support, and the challenge of continuing school, we offer intensive education and counseling for patients and their families.

Deliveries are referred to a nearby city hospital that has a midwife service with backup by an obstetrician. Barring complications, the mother and child return to the center two weeks after delivery. Initially these visits focus on postpartum care and physical exams for mother and child. As the child grows they encompass childhood immunizations and routine pediatric care. This continuity is one of the greatest rewards my work has to offer. I've followed some of these young families for years. It is hard to describe what I feel when I see babies whose mothers I cared for during pregnancy now walking, talking, and even going to school.

The most common chronic conditions we see include asthma (among children and adults), hypertension, diabetes, arthritis, and HIV infection. When therapy calls for a drug-based intervention, I have full prescriptive authority within the scope of family practice. This permits me to prescribe virtually any therapy that would be used in an ambulatory setting, including controlled substances such as Valium®, Demerol®, and phenobarbital. When appropriate, I counsel patients about nonpharmaceutical interventions. In this capacity, I might outline a program of behavior modification, including regular exercise and nutritional improvements.

As is true in many family practices, the acute illnesses we see usually take the form of ear infections, vaginitis, flu symptoms and strep throat, and sexually transmitted diseases. While most of these cases are no more or less than they appear to be, we are alert for the influence that domestic unrest, unemployment, or drug and alcohol abuse may be having in our patients' lives. In this respect, my practice gives me an advantage because the trust we have established enables us to know them and the events they experience. And because of our family orientation I may treat several generations or members of the same family. In a real sense, I become part of their lives.

Nonspecific acute symptoms such as recurring sore throats, headaches, sleeplessness, and body aches may be the product of a stressful life. I see inordinate stress among Hispanic women who feel oppressed by the traditional culture in which they live and were raised. They are torn between their ethnic loyalty and the freedom they see other women exercising in American culture. At times, their illnesses are manifestations of their frustration and troubling feelings. In such cases it is especially important to listen to patients and, perhaps, encourage them to set goals that can alleviate their distress. Some of these women I refer to our social worker or staff psychologist, who may be able to help them understand problems and find resources and solutions.

A small percentage of these nonspecific presentations go beyond circumstantial anxieties and cultural frustrations. Indeed, we see the victims of domestic violence, sexual abuse, and child abuse. In such cases, I ask patients directly if they have been beaten or abused. I ask point-blank questions about their drug use and family relationships. I make every effort to avoid guesswork and ambiguity. Regardless of what I discover, it is essential to remain nonjudgemental and to help my patients and their families work toward positive solutions.

For all the variety of conditions I encounter, I am able to provide appropriate care and intervention for roughly 90 percent of my cases. For the other 10 percent, I may consult with a staff physician, or I may need to refer the patient to a specialty physician.

In addition to my practice at the center, I am a faculty member at Columbia University's School of Nursing in New York. I teach an introductory course on primary care and a course on the applications of family systems theory in primary care nursing. I also am a preceptor for a clinical practice practicum. Although I enjoy the challenge of teaching, the practicum is special to me because of the opportunity it gives me for hands-on participation with students. Twice each week, students in a family nurse practitioner program gain clinical experience at the center by performing histories and physicals. I verify their physical findings and diagnoses and help them create plans for care. Not only is it exciting to watch the students gain confidence in themselves, but this contact also sharpens my own analytical skills.

One of the reasons I enjoy my practice so much is that the traditional relationship between doctors and nurses does not exist at the center. All of my colleagues are caring and supportive, and they all respect my capabilities. Equally gratifying are my patients, who are a constant source of spiritual triumphs. In the face of overwhelming odds, so many struggle to make changes in their lives — just staying in school or getting a job can be massively difficult in the Bronx. And the impact of AIDS has strained many families. For example, I recently cared for a woman with three children who lost her stable, loving husband to an illness that progressed very quickly. After his death, it was learned that he had AIDS, which he probably contracted as an IV-drug abuser prior to his marriage to my patient. Today, although the woman has tested positive, she continues her life with a dignity and serenity that I think few people could summon.

I don't mean to suggest that my practice is without frustrations. One of the most difficult of these is time limitations. Because I may see more than 20 patients in a day, I often am unable to spend as much time with each as I would like. Another frustration is that our limited resources allow us to serve only a small percentage of the people who need help in this neighborhood. Dealing with sickness and patients' personal lives is an intense experience that at times leaves me emotionally and physically exhausted. This can be tough on my own family.

Even so, the positive features of my career far outweigh the negatives. This practice offers a high degree of self-determination and mobility. Family nurse practitioners are in great demand in inner-city and rural areas; in many rural areas, the FNP may be the only health care provider for miles.

Certification in this specialty is provided by the American Nurses Association (ANA) and must be renewed every five years. Because of the depth of training they receive, certified family nurse practitioners also are qualified for positions as women's health nurse practitioners or pediatric nurse practitioners. Financially, this area of nursing is more rewarding than hospital-based practices and generally carries excellent benefits. In the New York City area, annual salaries for FNPs range from $40,000 to $80,000. Plentiful now, job opportunities probably will increase as the nation begins to place more emphasis on primary care.

There are a number of master's degree programs available for nurses with BSNs who are interested in primary care practice. Course requirements may vary between 30 and 60 credits. These programs provide extensive clinical training and involve hands-on practicums in clinical sites. They also have significant academic components, including instruction on disease states, disease processes, treatments, medications, family and patient education and counseling efforts, and health maintenance protocols. For nurses who lack a BSN, a few generic master's programs provide equivalent training. ANA certification is recommended for practice.

In my career as a family nurse practitioner I experience the satisfaction that goes with feeling I make a difference in my patients' lives. Each day I have opportunities to help people, ease their suffering, and encourage them to help themselves. Back when I decided that nursing met the criteria of my ideal job, I never imagined that it would turn out to be so much more than a job.

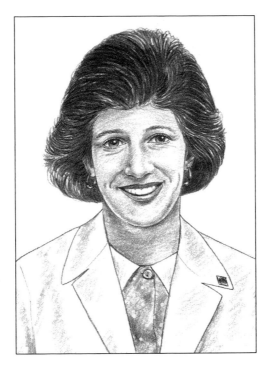

Kate Reilly Morency, MS, RN,C,
is a geriatrics nurse practitioner and a
nurse specialist at Beth Israel Hospital
in Boston, Massachusetts.

The Geriatrics Nurse Practitioner

I have always had a special place in my heart for older adults. Even when I was a child, some of my closest relationships were with people who were well over 60. But it took the insight and support of a head nurse for me to realize that my true talents lay in working with this patient population. Thanks to her, I have been able to create a fascinating practice.

In 1978, just after graduation from nursing school, I began practicing in a 28-bed general medical unit at Beth Israel Hospital in Boston. Beth Israel uses primary nursing as its professional practice model. In primary nursing, one nurse has 24-hour accountability for all the care a patient receives. Each nurse selects the patients she wishes to be the primary nurse for, and all patients are assigned a primary nurse within 24 hours after admission. After I had been at the hospital for about a year, my head nurse noticed that I was following a pattern in selecting the patients I wished to care for.

In my yearly evaluation we talked about the patients I had taken care of during the past 12 months. She wondered if I knew that I had consistently selected the oldest and sickest patients. I was shocked and said I had not realized it; I was just selecting the people I wanted to care for. I said I had always been drawn to the elderly and had grown up around older adults because many of our family friends were elderly. I had been very close to my grandparents and great-grandmother and thought older people were interesting. I also believed that because they were old, they might not get the care they needed. We talked a little longer and she asked if I would like to attend a workshop on caring for the elderly. I said yes, and that day-long session changed my life by giving my career new focus and clarity.

Presenters in the workshop talked about how most people in hospitals are old and have a very specific set of needs. They pointed out that the way illnesses manifest themselves in geriatric patients can vary dramatically from standard presentations. Moreover, because elderly bodies react differently to treatments and medications, the healing process does not necessarily result in expected outcomes. I was fascinated. At the time, geriatrics was a fairly new field, and I had not been exposed to these concepts.

By the end of the day I felt as though I were on fire. I knew then that geriatrics was meant to be the focus of my professional life. The very next day I looked into applying to graduate school, and in 1981 I received a master's in nursing and became certified as a geriatrics nurse practitioner. I spent the next two years at Beth Israel — the first in a geriatrics nurse fellowship, the second delivering specialized bedside care for seriously ill geriatric patients. I also was responsible for in-service education and training for staff nurses.

After that, I spent another year doing clinical research in a nursing home associated with the hospital and Harvard University's School of Medicine. Then, in 1984, I returned to the hospital to join a multidisciplinary geriatrics care team. I have been a member of this team ever since and have expanded my practice to include both inpatient and outpatient settings.

Inpatient responsibilities consume most of my practice time. Our team is diagnosis-specific, which means that we deal with a particular patient profile regardless of the unit. We are called in to see older adults who have problems that are beyond their unit's normal realm of care. For instance, a 90-year-old woman who was admitted to an orthopedic unit for a broken hip may now be presenting with a number of other conditions that the unit's staff believes can benefit from a consultation with someone who has expertise in geriatrics. These conditions can include depression, failure to thrive, delirium, and dementia. We also are called in to assess ethical issues, discuss proper use of drug therapy, or to provide opinions about whether it is safe for the patient to go home.

My team includes an attending physician, a geriatrics fellow, and a social worker. When we round, see new patients, meet with family members, and perform evaluations, all of us are present. This is an unusual approach, because on most other multidisciplinary teams, it is normal for members to perform their duties in their own time and for the entire team to meet, perhaps once a day, to discuss patients and findings. The condition of a geriatric patient can fluctuate quickly, and we decided in the beginning that it would be better for us and the patients if the team worked together. We reasoned that if we all see and hear the same things at the same time, the chances are good that we will be able to come up with better solutions to problems.

The team follows five to seven patients at a time. Our patients are usually over 85. Most are frail and extremely sick. Many are in the last year of life. Our evaluation of a new patient takes at least two hours of interview time. And before this meeting, team members spend even more time gathering information about the patient. For example, if he came here from a nursing home or was under the care of a visiting nurse, I will call the appropriate people to learn details of his daily care. Was he ambulatory? Did he experience episodes of delirium or disorientation? What medications was he on before his admission here? I also get in touch with the patient's family to learn what other factors we need to consider. Such detective work is time-consuming, but it gives us a much better grasp of the problem than simply going over the notes in the patient's chart. Besides, the team was formed to improve patient care, and the extensive background work we do is vital in accomplishing that mission.

During the face-to-face evaluation of patients, each team member examines and observes with a particular perspective in mind. I focus on functional status, not only in the current context, but also with the postdischarge environment in mind. Can patients ambulate and feed and dress themselves? How well are they capable of functioning? I also try to determine what nursing could do to make interactions with the patient more fruitful.

After the evaluation is completed, the team meets to discuss what we've seen and create a plan of care. We follow our patients until their problems are resolved or they are discharged. This includes daily follow-up visits to the patient's bedside that can take 15 minutes to half an hour. When possible, we like to have the primary nurse and the patient's family present because these people are a source of valuable information. For instance, if the patient has been disoriented or uncomfortable, a relative may be a better judge than we are about the effectiveness of our efforts. If our recommendations for treatment were unsuccessful, we discuss new alternatives with the primary nurse and keep family members informed of our efforts.

While our inpatient service is very comprehensive, it is not always cost effective. In some cases, we save money by solving problems that otherwise could extend the patient's length of stay. Our care also may prevent readmission. However, maintaining team members on the same schedule and allowing us to provide the kind of care we do is, at best, a break-even proposition for the hospital. In fact, this service exists only because our administration and staff have made a commitment to meet the special needs of our community's geriatric patients.

Our outpatient service is another way we address the needs of this population. The service was initiated by our department of gerontology to provide consultations for geriatric patients and their relatives who want second opinions or specialized advice. The service is staffed by me, two geriatricians, and a social worker. Some patients are referred to us by their physicians, some come on their own.

We had been performing outpatient geriatric evaluations informally for several years, because people often were not happy with their physicians, or because local physicians recognized that in some cases a geriatrics specialist might be better able to evaluate patients. As the demand became greater, we decided that it was time to establish a formal outpatient program.

As of now, this service provides consultation and limited primary care. Whether a patient is self-referred or sent by a physician, we prefer a physician's letter of introduction as well as past medical records and history. We ask that patients be accompanied by family members, a visiting nurse, or anyone else who participates in their day-to-day care. As with inpatients, all four team members make a comprehensive, head-to-toe evaluation.

Consultations are requested in order to address specific problems, many involving medications, which is one of our areas of expertise. Many of the patients we see believe they are being overmedicated or are concerned about adverse reactions. In truth, it is not uncommon for geriatric patients to visit their physicians complaining of a problem and come away with a new prescription—even though their problem may be a result of their current medications. These problems arise because many caregivers—nurses as well as physicians—fail to realize that the physiology of older people is very different from that of the average adult. Consequently, what protocols consider a normal adult dose is in no way a normal geriatric dose. For example, I once had a patient who had been prescribed medication to control his agitated nighttime behavior. However, when he took the medication, he became even more agitated. It turned out that while the prescription was well within the dosage range for a normal adult, it was 10 times stronger than we would recommend for a geriatric patient.

Along with medication problems, we see cases involving memory loss, incontinence, night wanderings, and severe arthritis. We also have visits from healthy older adults who want to know what preventive measures can help them remain healthy and maintain their quality of life. No matter what a patient presents with, I try to determine whether the problem is correctable or treatable. Any recommendations we make are forwarded to the patient's primary physician. Our outpatient service usually is provided in one or two visits, with the family calling in for further information—especially if we have recommended a series of tests or a change in drug therapies.

Nurses who want to forge a career in a geriatrics practice first need two to five years of experience in a general medical setting. During that time it would be advisable to take advantage of special geriatrics workshops and continuing education offerings. As you begin to assess master's degree programs, consider that some institutions offer combination programs in adult and geriatric care, while others focus strictly on geriatrics.

Choosing an institution is important, too. Many nurses have a general idea of what they want to do with their professional lives, but for the nurse who is fresh out of school and working in that very first job, just getting through the day takes a good bit of effort. So select your first job with care, looking for an institution that will provide a nurturing environment in which you can focus on your career goals as well as your daily responsibilities. In fact, I know the route I took to this practice would have been much more difficult had my first head nurse not taken the time to recognize my interests and give me encouragement. That type of support has been repeated in different ways during every step of my career here.

You will find many rewards in geriatrics, but for me, the greatest satisfaction lies in small things. Providing an intervention that can ease someone's pain or help a patient regain restful sleep may lack the drama of helping with an organ transplant, but to most of my patients, it is the little things that count. Many elderly people have grown accustomed to being shunted aside by the system, and they are grateful when someone takes time to care about their quality of life. Being able to help these patients is my greatest satisfaction.

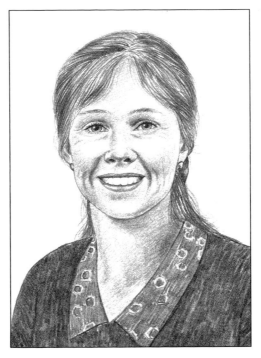

*Betty Jennings, MS, RN, CNM,
is in private practice with Colorado Nurse
Midwives and has faculty affiliation with the
University of Colorado Health Sciences
Center School of Nursing
Nurse Midwifery Program.*

The Nurse Midwife

Every woman's birth experience is different, and that's the way it should be. Unfortunately, traditional obstetric care doesn't always acknowledge that. Instead, there often is a presumption that pregnancy in itself is risky, and the resulting care can be restrictive and unfulfilling for the mother, her family, and the nurse. However, in the late 1960s and early 1970s, the women's movement began encouraging women to reject the high-technology approach to obstetric care and seek their own personal experiences. This shift in attitude opened up opportunities for nurses who wanted to practice midwifery. Today, as a nurse midwife, I have a practice that focuses on providing safe, satisfying care for mother and baby.

In 1965, I received my BSN from the University of Missouri in Columbia, and my master's degree in maternal-child nursing from the University of California, San Francisco, in 1969. While I had a theoretical background in maternity and family care, my master's focus was on the growth and development of the child, and my subsequent professional experience centered on pediatric nursing. After I graduated, I worked in an ICU at the St. Louis Children's Hospital, then as a bedside nurse at a hospital in Sun Valley, Idaho. It was in that job, where I had no particular specialty, that my interest in obstetrics was sparked. I realized that whenever there was a woman in labor, I wanted to take care of her.

Next I took a job as a junior instructor at the University of Oregon School of Nursing, teaching medical and surgical nursing. I also spent time on a hospital ship, the SS *Hope*, during its tour to Tunisia. After that I spent a couple of years teaching pediatrics to undergraduates at the St. Louis University School of Nursing. Finally, in 1972, I decided to move to Denver, to accept a job as the head nurse in the University of Colorado Health Sciences Center's University Hospital nursery.

It was there that I started thinking seriously about nurse midwifery. I saw tremendous resources devoted to the intensive care nursery. Everything was focused on sick infants, but I knew that we could keep many children out of the ICU if we could enhance the health care given to pregnant women. In the process we could improve pregnancy outcomes. By paying more attention to nutrition, substance abuse, and pregnancy planning, many adverse effects could be mitigated. It was clear to me that we needed to concentrate on preventive, health-oriented, continuous prenatal care.

Another nurse I worked with at the time had created a structure for labor and delivery nurses that not only put them on call for labor, but also involved them in ambulatory care before and after the delivery. That concept dovetailed with the mother-infant care we were delivering in a postpartum setting. As I began to study nurse midwifery, I discovered that the roots of continuity of care were born in its approach to labor and delivery.

In my next job, I worked with a nurse midwife who taught me the basics of prenatal care, including how to assess the growth and development of a baby, how to order and interpret lab evaluations, and how to identify early signs of complications. This woman was providing comprehensive prenatal care, but was not delivering babies. At that time, efforts were underway to make it legal for nurse midwives to deliver babies in Colorado. Thus, in 1975 I entered a South Carolina-based certification program for nurse midwives, confident that I could return to Denver and practice nurse midwifery from prenatal care through delivery to postpartum care.

Now, most certification programs are organized in conjunction with master's degree studies, but I was in a one-year, certification-only program that emphasized clinical training. Students worked in several clinics, providing care to clients that included inner-city women as well as those who came from poor, rural black communities with strong cultural traditions, extended family support, and few inner-city problems.

In addition, the nurse midwives on the faculty practiced in the community with women who sought out midwifery care, but were neither poor nor underserved; they were simply looking for alternative birthing care.

When I returned to Denver, I joined another nurse midwife and together we taught in an educational program for nurse practitioners at the University of Colorado Health Sciences Center. As a nurse midwife, I was thoroughly experienced in the training we were giving the nurse practitioners. In fact, nurse midwives are qualified to work as nurse practitioners in women's health and family planning. At the same time, we began laying the groundwork for a nurse midwifery educational program.

In 1978, my colleague and I began practicing midwifery at the University of Colorado Health Sciences Center Hospital. There we each worked 60 to 70 hours a week, providing comprehensive care. In our first year we delivered nearly 80 babies in addition to our faculty responsibility.

In 1980, we had convinced the university to establish a nurse midwifery training program, and our faculty increased to handle the academic responsibilities associated with teaching graduate students. Today, I'm still employed by the school of nursing, and I have a faculty practice with hospital privileges. Although I relinquished my official academic role when I became a mother myself, I am still informally involved in teaching.

In 1983 we extended our practice to a private hospital. The facility was ideal. For one thing, its nurses supported the concepts of midwifery. Many were older nurses who had extensive experience with less technological approaches to maternity care and were more receptive to the idea of natural childbirth. One nurse in particular supported our program and became influential in setting policy. She helped create an environment in which pregnant women could individualize their delivery. In this setting, laboring women are encouraged to ambulate. There's a Jacuzzi in every room, and families are welcome during labor and delivery. Assuring the well-being of the mother and baby during labor and birth can be accomplished while helping the women and family have the kind of birth experience they prefer. We stay with the woman and her family during labor and birth, and we also see her postpartum. After delivery, there are no strict visiting hours after which the baby must be returned to the nursery. In short, there are not a lot of restrictive routines. In fact, St. Luke's was the first hospital in the community to combine labor, delivery, recovery and postpartum care in single-room maternity care.

I still practice at the same hospital, which handles slightly less than 200 births a month — 10 percent of which are delivered by nurse midwives. The medical consultation for our practice is provided by an OB/GYN group with which we have a specific contractual agreement.

In my practice, most of my patients come through self-referral; they are women who are looking for an alternative to their current or previous care. Many find my practice in the Yellow Pages or are referred by a previous client. I work part time, some 20 hours a week. I'm in the office one or two days a week, and I'm on 24-hour call seven or eight days a month. While some nurse midwives are able to carve out practices that involve only shift work, many end up being on call, working nights and weekends. That, of course, comes with the territory.

When I'm in the office, many of the women I see have come in for introductory visits. Some are not even certain they want to use a nurse midwife. So, in our preliminary meeting I explain my education and role preparation, the care we deliver, and how our relationship with physicians works. Most nurse midwives provide care for healthy, low-risk women and are associated with an OB/GYN who manages problem patients. If a woman has complications in her pregnancy, we consult with a physician or arrange for the physician to examine the patient. Depending on the severity of the problem, we may transfer the patient into the physician's care. Often, we are able to continue to provide the component of nurse midwifery that includes support, education, and counseling, while the physician manages the complications. With a normal, uncomplicated pregnancy, it's entirely possible that the woman will never see a doctor.

Typically, I spend an hour and a half with a woman on her first visit. I take a history, perform a physical examination, and discuss her pregnancy. We talk about diet and exercise, we talk about preparation for pregnancy and birth, and we may discuss parenting issues. Although we don't teach our own childbirth classes, we do encourage women to enroll. Some women are well read and educated about childbirth; others need a great deal of information. After two weeks, I see the client again to go over her lab results. If there's a problem — from a cold to a bladder infection — I see her more often. In addition, many of my clients come back for annual exams. Sometimes, I provide counseling for women who plan to get pregnant.

The differences between care offered by a nurse midwife and an OB/GYN depend largely on the individual. In general, though, midwives concentrate more on continuous, preventive care. Not only do we address a woman's physiological condition, but we also consider the impact pregnancy will have on her family. During pregnancy, health not only means absence of medical complications, it also has to do with nutrition, exercise, rest, and psychosocial needs. I don't like to use the term *holistic care*; but I would say that through education and a strong commitment to prenatal care, nurse midwives meet the broader needs of women in pregnancy. We have a tradition of focusing on the mother's role, as she then can provide a healthy environment for her children.

One thing that's categorically different in the care provided by obstetricians and by midwives is that the nurse midwife is with the woman during labor — a physician generally is there only for delivery. We, along with the labor and delivery nurses, are the ones who rub the mother's back during contractions. I may take breaks to eat or take a nap, but often I'm there well after the labor and delivery nurse's shift has ended. Midwives share the entire birthing experience.

This can lead to professional jealousy. If a woman has been seeing an obstetrician, the labor and delivery nurses deliver care during labor. Because nurse midwives are so involved in labor, the hospital nurses may feel that we've deprived them of the heart of their job. It's very important that nurse midwives be sensitive to such feelings and work hard to maintain an effective professional relationship.

Before entering practice, a nurse midwife must find medical backup, enlist the support of a hospital, and be aware of the possibility for professional conflict. As can labor and delivery nurses, physicians can hamper a midwife's professional activities; they usually hold decision-making positions on hospital credentialing committees. Unless they work in settings where the value of their work is recognized, nurse midwives may well find themselves fighting uphill battles and struggling for respect.

That situation is improving, and nurse midwives are gaining a professional footing. In the community where I live, there are at least a dozen nurse midwives in private practice. Many of them were my students. As are all nurse midwives, they are qualified to provide preventive health care to women. Studies have proven the quality of their care and their cost effectiveness and demonstrate the satisfaction of their patients. In underserved populations, the improved outcome of births has been documented. We've seen reduced incidences of prematurity, reduced percentages of small-for-dates babies, and reduced infant mortality rates. The biggest issues facing nurse midwives right now have to do with filling our place in the overall scheme of health care reform.

Nurse midwifery offers an appealing combination of practice and teaching in a variety of settings: the office, the hospital, the acute care setting. In my work, I deal constantly with issues in gynecology, pregnancy, family planning, parenting, and public health. I have contact with patients, graduate students, nursery and labor and delivery nurses, pediatricians, neonatologists, obstetricians, and perinatal clinicians. My challenge is to tailor care specifically to individual women and their families. Nurse midwifery is a field with so much variety that it is hard to imagine being bored. It offers nurses autonomy and a chance to apply their skills, knowledge, and judgement. Just as a successful physician must, I've earned my clients' confidence and appreciation. I'll never see one of them looking over my shoulder and saying, "You can't do that. You're a nurse."

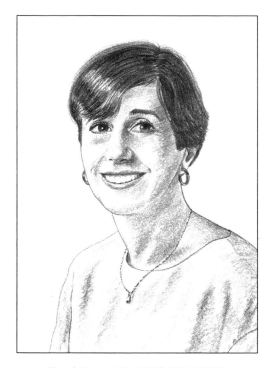

Carol Roye, MS, MEd, RN, CPNP,
is a pediatrics nurse practitioner in a
Manhattan school clinic that is affiliated with
Columbia Presbyterian Hospital,
New York, New York.

The Pediatrics Nurse Practitioner

Asthma and ear infections. Colds and congenital heart diseases. Sprained fingers and sexually transmitted diseases. Those problems are all in a day's work for me, a pediatrics nurse practitioner (PNP) in a New York City school-based clinic. Working with an underserved population, I am the health care point person for nearly 2,000 middle school children aged 11 to 15. For many, I am the primary health care provider.

For a number of years, I worked as a special education teacher (I have a baccalaureate degree in psychology and a master's in special education), then I quit to raise a family. In 1982, I decided to go back to work, but I didn't want to return to teaching. Instead, I opted to attend nursing school and entered a two-year master's program that was designed for students who already had a baccalaureate degree in another field.

I was trained to be a family nurse practitioner but realized later that I wanted to work only with children. As a result, I enrolled in a pediatric primary care program, another two-year master's program, which I completed in 1986. Since then I've become a certified pediatrics nurse practitioner.

After earning my degree, I took a job at a municipal hospital in the Bronx, working as a PNP in a clinic for teenage mothers and their babies. It soon became apparent to me that it's almost futile to work with young people unless their parents are included. So, in my five years at the clinic, I created a program specifically for the mothers of the teenagers I was seeing. The program's emphasis was on the importance of encouraging their daughters to use birth control and return to school.

Today, I'm studying the impact that program had on pregnancy and school attendance and on the quality of life for those young people. This study will become my dissertation for a doctoral degree in health education.

My work in the Bronx proved to be good training for my current practice. Here, we provide a complete range of medical services — from conducting physical exams to treating common illnesses and injuries. However, the basic intent of our efforts is to reduce the rate of pregnancy among students. Consequently, much of my time is spent on reproductive health care, treating STDs, and counseling about sexual activity and birth control. Because this clinic is in a middle school, we're not allowed to dispense birth control. We are able to refer students to appropriate sources.

One of our major challenges is dealing with children who are thinking about becoming sexually active. Generally, they are willing to talk openly and honestly about sex, and I find that after talking with me they are less likely to be impetuous. Discussing the risks and consequences in a clinical light has a way of diminishing the romance of sex.

Teenage sex happens for all kinds of reasons, and physical attraction often is low on the list. For some young people, sexual activity is an act of rebellion. And many girls feel that having a baby validates them in some way. For example, one 13-year-old girl I counseled was dating a boy who was quite a bit older. He wanted to have a baby, and she wanted to make him happy. However, she'd had a miscarriage before and was having trouble getting pregnant. She came to me for help.

In such situations, I emphasize the importance of making informed decisions about sex and pregnancy. I told this child that I understood the desire to have children, but I asked if she had weighed all the consequences of motherhood. For example, how would she finish her education? How would the two of them support the baby if neither had even a high school diploma? I also pointed out that young girls don't necessarily produce healthy babies; they're often born early and small. So, for that reason alone, I suggested that the best course might be to wait. The girl came to me several days later and said that not only had she decided against having a baby, she also had broken up with her boyfriend.

For every success like that one, there are times when it feels as though I'm beating my head against the wall. Particularly with psychological or sexual issues, the kids appear to understand what I'm telling them, but they still succumb to powerful social pressures. I may believe I've convinced a girl about the importance of birth control, and then she becomes pregnant. As frustrating as that can be, I've slowly learned that I can only do my best.

The word is out around school that it is okay to come to the clinic, and we have kids sending their friends in. We're never judgemental, and we respect the students' privacy. We do urge children to go to their parents with problems, but we don't violate their confidence unless the child's life is in danger.

Unfortunately, some of our students have severe emotional problems. In fact, every Friday from May until the end of school last year, someone made a suicide attempt. No one succeeded, but some of the children were in intensive care for days. Depression can be such a problem, and I try to identify emotionally disturbed students during routine histories, asking questions about whether the child has ever considered suicide and what the circumstances were. They're remarkably honest in answering, and I immediately refer at-risk children to a social worker.

On any given day, I have three or four kids scheduled for physical exams. I actually perform only two or three, because I can usually count on at least one not to show. I also ask students to come in for follow-up visits, and I treat walk-ins who have been injured in gym class, those scratched up in fights, or some who just have a cold or sore throat. All in all, I believe I see more significant health problems than the average pediatrician, probably because my students have had such poor medical care — if they've had any at all. Fairly serious congenital health problems, orthopedic anomalies, and vascular and endocrine disorders are not uncommon in our clinic.

Asthma, which is common among our mainly Hispanic population, is a significant problem here. In fact, it causes a good bit of absenteeism because the only care many of our asthmatic students receive is in the emergency room; chronic management is an abstract concept in most cases. Fortunately, asthma can usually be kept under control, and when I am aware of its presence I'm able to intervene to minimize repeat attacks. Moreover, because I'm based in a school I can manage care effectively because I don't have to depend on parents to bring their kids in for an appointment. Also, I can write prescriptions (asthma medications and antibiotics are the most common) and order lab tests if necessary.

In addition to medical concerns, I must pay attention to the family situations our students live in. For instance, it is important for me to know if I am dealing with a mother who can remember to give her child medicine three times a day. Another of the PNP's responsibilities is to help parents understand what behaviors are normal in their children. I let them know that the sometimes unpleasant aspects of living with an adolescent are not only normal, but they actually are necessary manifestations of the transition from adolescence to maturity.

Beyond my clinic duties, I teach in Columbia's PNP graduate program, and I precept students in the hospital nursery and at a nearby nursery school. We have a special nursery for infants who cannot go home with their mothers, usually because we've found drugs in the baby's urine. Naturally, we must keep the baby until its urine is clear, but evidence of drug use raises larger questions about safety in the home. It also raises the spectre of AIDS and exposure to other diseases. My students work with these babies, because the mother is not waiting anxiously, and the babies benefit from the extra attention.

In interviewing a mother to determine whether the home is a safe and appropriate environment in which to raise an infant, the PNP asks very basic questions: Is there a crib at home? Do you plan to breast feed? If not, do you have formula at home? If the PNP has any concerns, a social worker becomes involved in making a collaborative decision about whether the baby should go home. In such cases, the final decision is made by the social worker, not the nurse.

Working at the nursery school can be an eye-opening experience. The children there all have been required to have preschool physical examinations, but we frequently diagnose serious problems, including heart murmurs, abdominal masses, teeth erosion, and visual acuity problems that have been missed by the pediatrician.

Traditionally, pediatrics nurse practitioners have worked in outpatient settings with underserved populations, but there are other practice options to consider as well. For instance, more and more newborn nurseries are being staffed by PNPs. Other practice settings for PNPs include freestanding or hospital-based outpatient clinics and mobile vans that deliver health care in certain communities. Another trend in the field is for PNPs to follow patients after they have been admitted to the hospital. This is an ideal way to deliver care, because the PNP knows the patient better than the staff does.

In any setting, a PNP who can't deal with a problem must feel comfortable asking for medical backup. No one gets upset if nurses ask for help when it's needed. However, lots of people get upset if advice is not sought when it should have been.

In some cases, pediatricians call a PNP for a second opinion. In fact, I recently had a call from a pediatrician who had examined a girl's cervix and was worried because it didn't appear normal. Because I have considerable experience in this area and have written articles about the adolescent cervix, it was reasonable for her to seek my expert opinion. In other words, the lines that delineate the roles of pediatricians and pediatrics nurse practitioners are blurring. Indeed, some 80 to 90 percent of what a pediatrician does can be done by a nurse practitioner. Consequently, as the U.S. health care system begins to rely more on primary care providers, pediatricians may be called on to address complex health problems, while PNPs deliver primary care.

However, specialization is not uncommon in this field, and a growing number of PNPs specialize in outpatient care for HIV-positive patients. I deal exclusively with adolescents, and others work only with hematologic or developmental problems. And when the pediatrics nurse practitioner combines traditional nursing skills (eg, communicating and teaching) with advanced physical assessment and diagnostic skills, the opportunities for a challenging career are virtually unlimited.

Several significant issues confront the pediatrics nurse practitioner. One that we've just resolved in New York State is prescription privileges — we now can prescribe narcotics. One issue we have yet to resolve is third-party reimbursement. Another is that with the national directive for changes in health care that would tie everyone into managed care, it is unclear what would happen to the school-based clinic; for many kids, we are the first line of defense.

From infants to teenagers, my practice contains the broadest possible range of activity. And there is never any doubt about the value of my efforts — I *know* what a difference I can make in the lives of my patients. How could there be greater professional rewards than those I receive in helping children who really need my care?

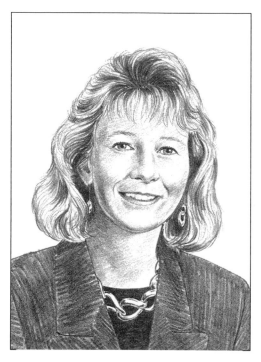

Carol Mest, MSN, RN,C,
was executive director of OccuMed Resources,
in Bethlehem, Pennsylvania,
at the time of the interview.
She is now the administrator of the
Centers for Occupational Health,
Crozer-Keystone Health System,
Media, Pennsylvania.

The Occupational Health Nurse

Several years ago, I learned that my father has asbestos disease — a result of his employment in shipyards. Fortunately, he's not seriously ill, but his situation strikes a very personal chord in my work, and it was a major factor in my decision to enter this field.

I'm the executive director of a company that contracts to provide occupational health services to several companies in the area. We visit these sites regularly to care for their employees. These and several other companies use our clinic on an as-needed basis.

After a false career start in biology, I realized that working in a lab isn't really my cup of tea. I wanted contact with people and believed that nursing would give me that while addressing my interest in science. In 1980, I received a BSN and went to work at the Hospital of the University of Pennsylvania. During my tenure there, I met a nurse practitioner who was performing a preoperative physical on one of my patients. This was the first nurse practitioner I had ever met, and we talked extensively about her work. I was quite interested, so I went over to the school of nursing to find out about the programs it offered. By then, the practitioner movement had been around awhile, but I don't think anyone realized how important it was to become.

In 1982 I started work on my master's degree in the University of Pennsylvania's nurse practitioner program. My emphasis was on adult care, and I finished my degree in 1984. During my studies, I did clinical work in an HMO and in a city-funded health clinic. After graduating, I accepted a job running a student health center. During the summer I worked in a clinic that had been established to serve migrant farm laborers. We treated the workers for injuries sustained during work, and we offered their families a full range of social services. That was my introduction to occupational health care.

Most of our patients were poor young men from Mexico. One man told me he had walked from Mexico, and it wasn't hard to believe because these men didn't come to us in the healthiest state. We saw a range of occupational injuries: sprains, back strains, fractures, inhalation of pesticides, dermatitis, and repetitive-motion disorders. Also, many of the men were single, drank heavily, and used prostitutes — and they also suffered the consequences.

Back then, occupational health was not a burning issue for those who employed our patients, and I spent a lot of time marketing our services. We met with growers and farm owners to discuss the health care services their workers needed. We also turned to the community:

If a patient needed to visit a specialist, we solicited local organizations for funds. My duties also included providing transportation and translation services.

I became so interested in the Latino population that in my current PhD work in health education I'm writing a dissertation on how social support affects pregnancy outcomes in Latino women.

In the late 1980s, I came to work in this hospital-based occupational health program that provides on-site services to local companies. Our local economy is dominated by regulated industries in manufacturing and transportation. Most have between 200 and 300 employees, and while a few have physicians who treat injuries and perform pre-employment physicals, most do not have medical professionals who work proactively to identify hazards in the workplace and prevent injuries.

By starting with a couple of smaller companies, we gained entree into the tougher clients. Now, we work with about 10 companies, providing the services of registered nurses and nurse practitioners in four-hour to 20-hour blocks of time. The nurse visits the company to treat injuries or illnesses, do follow-up visits, provide medical surveillance and testing, and to institute prevention and screening programs.

At the start of our relationship with a client, we usually ask to see the last three years of workers' compensation claims, and then we do a detailed analysis of that information. We categorize injuries according to body part, nature and severity, the department in which it occurred, the task being performed when it was sustained, the amount of time lost due to the injury, and the amount of money it cost. We speak with the attending physician and the insurance carrier, and then we inspect the plant, interviewing employees. I don't want a supervisor or plant manager to tell me what Joan does on the knitting machine. I want Joan to show me. If an employee is in pain, I want him or her to tell me — many don't complain to management for fear of losing their jobs.

One of our clients manufactures customized glass. When we began working with the company, my assessment of the plant revealed a lot of complaints about the physical set-up. Many work stations were arranged so employees had to reach too far for supplies and frequently tripped over things because the area was too crowded. People who worked in painting areas reported that they developed rashes and sometimes felt dizzy or light-headed, probably a result of poor ventilation. In addition, there was no official quota system, but productivity records maintained subtle pressure on employees.

Using this information, we established certain goals, which we prioritized according to the simplicity of solving a problem and the severity of potential consequences if the problem was not addressed quickly.

Good housekeeping is basic to safety in any workplace, so we re-arranged the production area at the glass company in order to reduce dangerous clutter. In one situation, we proposed a policy of rotating job activities every two hours. This significantly cut the incidence of carpal tunnel syndrome. As is true throughout nursing, accomplishing our goals involved considerable education and reinforcement.

At another client company, a 200-employee lumber mill, workers were being injured at a rate of four or five per day. Drawing on my own emergency room experience, I met with the hospital administrator, and together we wrote a letter to the plant's manager, explaining that we suspected problems in the workplace and would like to meet with him to see if we could help. The manager took us on a tour, and I noticed that rules requiring the use of safety equipment were not being enforced. The safety glasses, face shields, and ear protectors that should have been standard equipment simply weren't being faithfully used. And, even though a company is liable for a workers' compensation claim, some employers are reluctant to be strict with employees who don't want to wear the gear. I made two recommendations. One was to make using protective equipment a condition of employment. The other, which the supervisor preferred, was to make an employee's safety record—including use of safety gear—part of his performance evaluation. Thus, failure to take appropriate safety precautions would directly influence pay increases. The supervisor's rationale was that if his company was not a safe business, it might as well not be in business at all, and employees who weren't working safely could not be rewarded. He reasoned that if safe practices were tied to a paycheck, compliance levels would rise.

One of the companies we work with identified problems independently and called us to help solve them. Company executives were expecting the government to institute an ergonomic standard and wanted to get a head start on meeting it.

I spent hours inspecting the factory, talking with employees, videotaping their movements, and even performing some of their job activities myself. Then I sat down with supervisors and managers to explain what needed to be done. I had them fill out a rather detailed questionnaire: What is the plant layout? Are there complaints from employees about work activities? Do workers complain that their jobs require too much twisting and moving? Do they report numbness or tingling in their fingers? Which jobs in the plant are highly repetitive? Are employees required to rotate their duties? Once I had a feel for the situation, I was able to use such information in setting priorities for what needed to be done. Then I moved to the more personal level of interviewing employees about their work. After that, we began to implement specific solutions.

Sometimes a bureaucratic structure can hinder very simple solutions. For instance, I work with a company whose workers belong to a union. Their contract stipulates that job rotation is not allowed. However, I suspect using that as an excuse wouldn't go over too well with OSHA, so I encouraged this client to try to renegotiate its union contract.

I work with clients in a variety of industries, from chocolate to cold storage, from textiles to trucking. Truck drivers have very particular problems. Truck cabs vibrate and bounce, and climbing in and out of them can be difficult. Combine those conditions with the profile of a typical truck driver: someone who's constantly on the road, smokes, has bad nutrition, and sleeps irregularly. This person has a pretty tough lifestyle that can inspire a host of health problems, not the least of which are hemorrhoids, kidney problems, and back injuries. Also, because of their schedules, it's difficult to get truck drivers to come in for care. Consequently, I schedule exams as early as 6:30 in the morning. I go far beyond Department of Transportation requirements, because I know my efforts may well be the only health care these workers get.

Traditionally, occupational health nurses are thought of as people who work in a dispensary, handing out aspirin and taking blood pressures. That's an old notion. The new reality is that we are extremely proactive. Rather than spending our time sitting in offices, we make plant inspections and conduct seminars. I might initiate a smoking-cessation program, then contract with a physician to come in with a presentation on the value of nicotine patches. I've addressed issues for substance abuse and mental health, and I've been responsible for motivational and personal growth seminars.

In the glass company I described earlier, many of the employees with whom I work are young, single mothers. For these workers, I address women's health concerns. And even though some subjects aren't directly related to occupational health, I talk about parenting, general wellness, even finances — global issues that profoundly affect these women's lives.

Because of the skills and background required in occupational health, this is an ideal practice for a nurse practitioner. But to do it well, nurses must be able to talk with the lowest-level employee, then turn around and translate his concerns into a bottom-line issue that the most senior manager can appreciate. Occupational health nurses must switch hats in a heartbeat, and not everyone can do that. For those who can, it's a wonderful job.

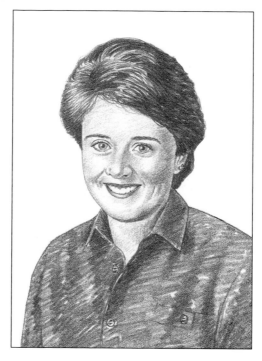

Trish McGovern, MSN, RN, OCN,
is an advanced practice nurse in oncology at
Columbia Presbyterian Medical Center,
New York, New York.

The Oncology Nurse

Nobody wanted to work on the oncology unit. That's what I discovered while working summers during college as a nursing assistant at my community hospital. The prevailing mentality was that everyone in oncology was dying, so the student nurses would plead with each other to switch assignments. Because I had worked at a nursing home in high school, I had experienced people dying. It didn't frighten me. In fact, it rather interested me. So when I was asked to switch with someone, I didn't mind.

I was working toward my BSN degree and by my senior year I knew I wanted to specialize in oncology nursing. I graduated in 1985 and took a position as a staff nurse at Columbia Presbyterian Medical Center (CPMC) in the adult research oncology unit. I've been here ever since. The most important lesson I have learned in my time here is that the diagnosis of cancer is not synonymous with death. In fact, diagnosis, treatment, and the management of treatment side effects have improved so much that many types of cancer are potentially curable.

I worked nights my first year at CPMC, days for the next, and in 1987 I became the assistant head nurse of the oncology unit. Then in 1988, I entered the master's degree program at Columbia University School of Nursing. Late in 1990, the hospital created a new position, oncology nursing clinician, which I held until September of 1993. I completed my master's of science in nursing (MSN) in oncology in the spring of 1991. In addition, I am an oncology-certified nurse. For someone considering oncology nursing, I strongly recommend a BSN program, followed later by an MS degree and certification. And for an advanced practice role, such as a clinical nurse specialist (CNS) or nurse practitioner (NP) as a career goal, many good master's programs are available.

In our 36-bed unit we see many different types of cancer, from hematological malignancies, such as leukemia, to the solid tumors, including cancers of the breast, lung, prostate, and colon. At any given time, between 10 and 12 of our patients are there to receive scheduled chemotherapy. The rest have complications, including infections, pain, or side effects from their treatment.

Nurses here must go through a six-week orientation program, as well as an additional two-week course on the specialized aspects of oncology nursing, which mainly have to do with administering chemotherapy and managing its side effects. During this initial period, nurses spend about half their time in a classroom and the other half applying their knowledge and skills.

Each nurse in this unit is responsible for six to eight patients, including the administration of their chemotherapy. Before starting treatment, the nurse meets with the patient and explains what side effects may be expected and what the patient can do to minimize them. We describe problems that may develop, and we make sure that patients know when they should call the doctor. In an effort to minimize the occurrence of nausea or vomiting, the nurses usually administer antiemetic agents as ordered by the physician before starting IV chemotherapy. Once the treatment is over, the nurse monitors the patient for potential side effects. The nurses monitor urine output and fluid intake closely, to ensure that kidney damage from the drug is avoided.

To minimize problems during hospitalization and after discharge, the nurses have regular contact with attending physicians, resident staff, and social workers. Some patients are reluctant to ask questions of their doctors, and the nurses function as a backup to answer questions and reinforce clinical information. In that sense, we are important conduits. For example, even when they are in a great deal of pain, some patients are afraid to ask the doctor for more medication because they don't want to seem addicted. In truth, addiction is extremely rare among cancer patients, and it is the nurse's job to communicate the patient's needs to the physician and to teach the patient the difference between tolerance and addiction. The oncology nurse becomes the patient's advocate. A nurse spends eight or 12 hours with a patient and is in the best position to inform other members of the health care team about the patient's needs.

Pain management is one of the most challenging issues for oncology nurses. While medication is most effective, we also teach nonpharmaceutical approaches to pain management, including self-hypnosis, relaxation, and imaging techniques. These methods help maximize pain relief.

In oncology, psychosocial and family matters are just as important as medical issues. Most patients go through different emotional stages when given the diagnosis of cancer. These stages include grieving, anger, denial, bargaining, depression, and acceptance. Some never get past the anger, and some never work through the depression. Some have bad days and regress temporarily. But most patients — and this is one of the reasons I find oncology nursing rewarding — find the inner strength to deal with their conditions. They are confronting the possibility of dying, and they fight against it. Or, realizing that they can't win the battle, they struggle to improve the time they have left.

Almost every cancer patient goes through an emotional crisis, and some need help moving from panic to a practical state of mind. As a nurse, I try to determine what coping strategies, resources, and support systems are available to the patient. Will the patient have trouble taking care of himself or getting around? How much impact will the disease have on his quality of life? Are family members available to help? We hold weekly education and support group meetings and encourage patients and their families to ask questions about their disease, treatments, and side effects. We discuss how they can cope with changed family roles and help them find ways to keep control over their lives.

Frequently the issue of insurance comes up. This hospital is in a lower socioeconomic area, and we often care for homeless patients or people without insurance or without enough insurance to cover the care they need. One of the worst parts of this job is seeing a patient become impoverished because he is ineligible for Medicaid, but unable to pay for his care and still be able to pay for rent, food, and other essentials.

We take care of many patients from diagnosis until cure and others through progression of disease and, finally, death. As a result, it's important for the oncology nurse always to know the stage of disease so we can prepare patients for what might happen in the future and adjust our goals accordingly. For instance, our goal with a new patient is to cure or control the disease. For patients with advanced cancer, our goal may change to palliation — managing symptoms such as pain and nausea and providing as much comfort as possible.

Typically, a newly diagnosed patient who is coming in for chemotherapy is frightened. At this point, the nurse's role is to minimize anxiety by answering questions and explaining what treatment will involve. One of my patients was a widower with children who lived far away. I was worried about the man's support system, and I knew he believed chemotherapy would be as terrible as his disease. All this had made him gruff and monosyllabic — a very angry man. I remained friendly and offered him openings to talk about his anxiety. Late one night when he was unable to sleep, I came in and asked if he wanted a sleeping pill and continued to talk to him. I made a number of open-ended statements such as, "You must be very frustrated." He began to vent his anger and his feelings of loss of control. Before long, he began to trust that I would give straight answers to his questions, and I was able to reassure him about some of the things he feared. By addressing his concerns, I was able to decrease his anxiety and give him the information he needed so that he felt more control over his situation.

As important as it is to offer a sympathetic ear, oncology nurses are highly susceptible to becoming personally involved with patients and their families — that's one thing to remain aware of. These patients are so eager to latch onto a comforting person that it's easy for the nurse to feel more like a member of the family than a professional. When a nurse deals with patients all day long, meeting their kids and taking responsibility for everything from their bodily functions to their emotional well-being, it's hard to not get attached. This happened to me several times before I realized I couldn't survive on such an emotional roller coaster. Losing those patients was like losing family members. Imagine doing that once every couple of months! Now, I have a sense of where that invisible boundary lies between the personal and the professional. I'll sit and talk with patients, and I'll get upset if they die. But I've adopted the philosophy that if I've made someone's illness easier to deal with, then I've done my job. But it is a priority to take care of my own emotional and physical well-being. If I don't do that first, I will not be effective in my job. Nurses who get so attached that they feel that they're never doing enough are headed for burnout.

Burnout is common in high-stress health care, but here we try to manage the problem by encouraging nurses to vent their feelings. We all know it's okay to go back to the lounge and get upset, and we often use lunch to brainstorm about a problem on the floor. Over time, we have become so sensitive to each other's thoughts that we can tell something is wrong by looking at a colleague's face.

All is not gloom and doom in the oncology unit. People do not die every day, and many do not die at all. It's hard to describe the elation nurses feel when their diligence keeps a leukemia patient out of the ICU and he goes into remission and can go home. Still, it's true that under our current health care system, more and more people are getting chemotherapy as outpatients, so the patients who are admitted are sicker. Sometimes, we have to remind ourselves that there are hundreds of people in the outpatient area who are cured of their cancer. Many of the patients we see in the hospital have more advanced disease.

An oncology nurse can elect to work at a cancer hospital where individual wards are dedicated to different types of cancer. Or, as I did, she or he might decide not to specialize in any particular area of oncology, choosing instead a hospital like Columbia Presbyterian, which has an oncology unit but treats other patients as well. Oncology nursing is not limited to hospital practice. Oncology nurses can be found in outpatient clinics, doctors' offices, or in home care agencies. They might be involved in cancer prevention or hospice care, and many participate in cancer screening and cancer prevention seminars. Those are all valid career choices for the oncology nurse.

There are opportunities for advancement in oncology nursing. Recently, I left the position of oncology nursing clinician to accept a new position as director of the Columbia Presbyterian Cancer Center Protocol Office. I am responsible for coordinating all clinical research data, working with our data managers, research nurses, and physicians. We are conducting cutting-edge research, testing new chemotherapy drugs for effectiveness and toxicity, and using autologous bone marrow transplantation against solid tumors such as breast cancer and brain tumors as well as other experimental treatments.

Not only is it exciting to be participating in medical research, I also have the opportunity and the resources to conduct clinical nursing research, to investigate better ways to manage side effects of treatment, and to meet the needs of patients and their families more effectively.

I have considered nursing in the ICU or ER, but I enjoy the challenges of oncology nursing. There always are new problems to be addressed, new approaches to be tried. And when a tough problem does crop up, I know that the oncology nursing staff will meet the challenge.

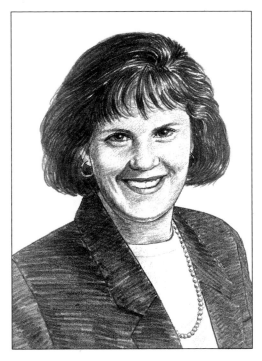

*Lisa Norsen, MS, RN,C,
is an advanced practice nurse in
cardiothoracic surgery at
Strong Memorial Hospital,
Rochester, New York,
and a senior associate in the
University of Rochester School of Nursing.
She precepts graduate students in the clinical
area and lectures on cardiac care in
the graduate program.*

The Cardiology Nurse

When I entered college, I had no intention of studying nursing, even though my mother was a nurse and a very positive role model for me. Growing up, I had spent endless hours talking with her about the profession and listening to stories about her work. I even spent several years as a patient care volunteer while I was a teenager. As far as I was concerned, I knew all about nursing. I wanted to be a biology teacher, and I spent most of my first two years in school studying toward that goal.

But sometime during my sophomore year it occurred to me that if I actually reached my goal, my career options would be fairly limited. The more I thought about this, the more it worried me. I could tell that I had changed a great deal in just a few semesters of college, and I imagined I might continue to do so. Consequently, I realized that I needed a career that would change with me as I went through life. This led me to think about other science-related majors. A faculty advisor suggested I consider nursing—the profession I thought I knew so much about. Nursing, she pointed out, has a strong science component. As I investigated further, I learned that the activities of nurses are not necessarily restricted to patient care, as I had always assumed. As a nurse I could teach, engage in research, become an administrator, or follow many other career paths. I had never understood the scope of the profession. Suddenly, it all clicked for me, and I made the best decision of my life: I transferred into the school of nursing.

In 1977, I graduated with a baccalaureate degree in nursing and went to work as a staff nurse in a surgical intensive care unit at Strong Memorial Hospital. I enjoyed caring for patients in this setting, and I liked the technological aspects of an ICU practice. The work was exciting—each day offered new challenges. After about a year, I decided I wanted to specialize, to assume a more autonomous role in patient care and to become active in research. This meant going back to school for a master's degree, which I completed in 1982. Soon after that, I began my career as an advanced practice nurse in cardiothoracic surgery.

A staff nurse is attached to a single patient care unit, but I belong to a multidisciplinary team that cares for all adult patients who will be undergoing cardiac surgery. I see these patients each day, following them from admission and preoperative care, through their surgery and postoperative rehabilitation. I also see them in an outpatient setting after discharge. I share this practice with two other advanced practice nurses. Our service is designed so that two of us are here between 6:30 AM and 7:00 PM, Monday through Friday. In general, we handle 20 patients at a time; the average length of stay is six to seven days.

My work begins when a patient is admitted to the hospital for cardiac surgery. I perform a preoperative assessment, which includes a physical exam and complete history. This helps me determine what medical and nursing therapies should be initiated before surgery and, to some extent, what we should plan on doing afterwards. I give each patient detailed information about the surgical experience. I explain what the procedure will be like, what the patient will feel and experience in the first few days after the surgery, and what goals the surgery is expected to achieve. During the preoperative phase, we also make sure the patient is thoroughly educated in lifestyle changes that can lower future risks. All of this is very important, because numerous studies have shown that patients have better surgical outcomes if they have been told what to expect beforehand. I am continually amazed at the number of patients who are admitted to the hospital without really understanding why. For example, many don't understand that bypass surgery is a treatment rather than a cure for heart disease.

When my patients go into surgery, so do I. This is part of the concept that underlies continuity of care. However, surgery is the crux of a patient's hospital experience, and I enjoy being there. I may participate in harvesting the saphenous vein—the vein used for bypass surgery—or I may be first in assisting the cardiac surgeon.

Not everyone is cut out to be in the OR. I like working there because it provides a very dynamic, collaborative experience involving surgeons, anesthesiologists, perfusionists, scrub nurses, perhaps a resident, and me. Most of the barriers come down in this environment where we all know our jobs and execute them in the most professional manner possible. I also enjoy doing procedures and working with the more technical aspects of surgery.

A bypass operation takes about four hours. If my job is to harvest the saphenous vein, I make the incision in the patient's leg, dissect the tissue away from the vein, and extract as much of the vessel as the surgeon needs. Then I suture the incision. After I am finished, I usually leave the OR and return for closing. If I am assisting, I stay for the whole procedure.

Postoperative management is probably the most involved part of my clinical practice because it comprises the majority of the patient's hospital stay. This care is based largely on our assessment of the patient's progress. We follow protocols that tell us what we should be seeing in recovery and how the patient should be progressing through the rehabilitation program. We compare these protocols with the patient's actual progress and alter therapy accordingly.

Throughout the postoperative process I pay special attention to patient education and counseling. It is important to remember that every patient is different and will have different responses, both physically and emotionally, to surgery. This means that I must collaborate closely with the nursing staff during this period. We each make our own assessments and then compare findings. The results will help us determine the best approach to care for each patient.

In an ideal scenario, the patient's progress follows every protocol. This means that all tubes and monitoring equipment — invasive and otherwise — are removed after the first day. The patient will get up and start to move around after day two. There will be no infections and no pulmonary, cardiac, or other complications. Also on day two, the patient starts watching video tapes about diet, exercise, and discharge activities. The schedule of activity, rehabilitation, and education will intensify gradually until the patient is discharged.

I examine each patient daily during rounds and, based on my findings, order appropriate medical therapies, medications, and tests. Pulmonary and cardiac complications are fairly common. Pulmonary complications usually manifest themselves in the form of atelectasis or plural effusions. Atelectasis (partial collapse of the lung) may be a result of the patient's dependency on the bypass machine during surgery. Plural effusions occur when a small amount of fluid collects along the outside of the lungs. Common cardiac complications include arrhythmias, fluid overload, and aberrations of serum electrolytes, the latter usually including reductions in potassium levels. When any complication occurs, my job is to manage the problem in order to prevent potentially serious sequelae. These complications usually can be resolved before discharge.

After discharge I follow patients through our outpatient department. After a week, I telephone their homes and conduct a progress survey. I ask questions that help me gauge how well they are doing: How are you feeling? Are you able to lie down comfortably at night? How do your sutures look? How is your appetite? Are you in pain? How far can you walk without experiencing shortness of breath? How do you believe you're doing? If the patient is having any problems, he or she is seen immediately in the outpatient department for an evaluation. Patients who are progressing well are scheduled to visit our outpatient clinic about three weeks after discharge. At that time, I conduct another interview and a physical examination. If everything looks fine, the patient continues rehabilitation under the care of his own physician.

Throughout this entire process, it is important to maintain interaction with the patient's family. Typically, I spend a significant amount of time counseling relatives and teaching them what they need to know about the patient's condition and about the kind of care he will need after discharge. If a patient does not do well after surgery, my contact with the family intensifies, and I become the link between the family and the medical team. I also become a conduit for counseling, support, and information. At times this can be emotionally draining, but nurses are uniquely able to perform these services. I wouldn't want to be a nurse if this component was missing from my practice.

In addition to my clinical duties, I coordinate the nurse practitioner group in surgery. This requires that I do program orientation for new nurse practitioners and make annual performance evaluations. Beyond that, I help plan projects for the group, such as sponsoring conferences on patient care, developing patient education materials, and organizing professional development seminars.

Strong Memorial Hospital supports the scholarly pursuits of advanced practice nurses because the administrators know that research, publishing, and presentations help improve the quality of patient care. I really enjoy research, and my involvement in it has grown considerably over the past few years. Most recently, I was the principal investigator on a study that examined the efficacy of progressive muscle relaxation and imagery in the management of postoperative pain. We taught a group of patients how to use cognitive skills that could help them relax and control their pain. We are still analyzing the data, but we believe the study will yield positive results. If it does, we will begin teaching those skills to all postoperative patients.

Can you imagine the excitement of participating in a project that leads to better patient care — and then being able to put the results into practice? Once the data have been analyzed, the information will be more available to all health care professionals through presentations at meetings and publication in journals. This recognition is a very satisfying part of the advanced practice role. And that I have been able to increase my own involvement in research while maintaining a clinical practice is yet another example of how I have been able to adapt my practice to my interests.

When I count the time I spend in my clinical practice, administrative duties, research, and educational efforts, there is little left for other interests. I could take hours from my personal life, but my leisure time and the time I spend with my family is treasured. Besides, it is essential to get away from my practice in order to recharge my batteries. In any case, if there were more hours in my professional day, I am sure I would find a way to spend them.

The advanced practice cardiac care nurse functions in a dynamic environment that demands highly refined skills. At least two years of staff experience in critical care is requisite, and so is a master's degree and certification as an acute care nurse practitioner. In this specialty, success — and patients' lives — depend on self-confidence and excellent critical thinking, as well as decision-making skills. Indecisive people need not apply.

No matter what type of practice you choose, nursing offers an advantage that no other health care profession can provide: adaptability. Simply put, our profession is uniquely able to accommodate a nurse's aspirations and interests. My own career is proof of this. I was drawn into nursing by my desire to teach and provide patient care. As I became interested in cardiac care I was able to refocus my practice in that direction. And now, I am augmenting my research endeavors by pursuing a PhD in nursing. With each step, I have been able to shape my career to fit my life, instead of the other way around. As a result, my career has never been less than fresh and exciting.

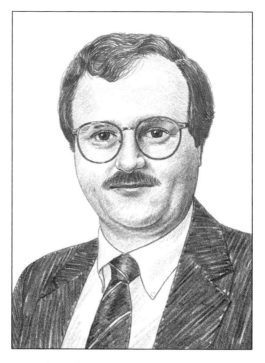

Patrick Coonan, MEd, MPA, RN,
is assistant director of nursing and director
of the Center of Emergency Training
and Development at
North Shore University Hospital,
Manhasset, New York.
He also is director of the critical care
graduate program at
Columbia University School of Nursing,
New York, New York.

The Emergency Room Nurse

We call it "the big save," because in the emergency department, that's the name of the game. It's like being in the bottom of the ninth inning with the score tied. The ball is hit into the outfield, and the centerfielder runs three steps up the wall to catch it and save the day. The big save is the best part of being an emergency department nurse, and I've done it for 15 years.

I spent the first 10 of those years in inner-city emergency departments in the Bronx and Harlem. Then in 1987 I made a dramatic career change and accepted the position of assistant director of nursing at North Shore University Hospital in affluent, suburban Long Island.

I had a tentative interest in pharmacy after high school, but one semester in pharmacy school convinced me that it wasn't for me. Instead of continuing with college, I withdrew and became a volunteer fireman and an emergency medical technician for a private ambulance company. It took a couple of years for me to realize that I couldn't go through life making five dollars an hour. So when a friend suggested I consider nursing, it occurred to me that such a career would not only allow me to continue helping people, it would also enable me to make a solid living. I entered a four-year BSN program.

After graduation I went to work as an emergency department nurse at a 600-bed teaching hospital in the Bronx. In those days, my background as an advanced EMT qualified me to start in the ED. Now, New York State law requires new graduates to gain at least a year's experience in another setting.

Every emergency department reflects the socioeconomics of its area, and inner-city emergency nursing can be quite an introduction to health care. Patients present with gunshot wounds, stab wounds, and drug overdoses. Pregnant women deliver in the emergency department. Children come in with illnesses that could have been prevented with proper immunization. For the urban poor, the ED serves as the family doctor and the community center, and one of the biggest challenges is dealing with the patients' social conditions.

Some patients come in feigning chest pains, simply to get a little human contact and evidence of concern. In such cases, I take a few minutes to chat. And, making sure patients understand discharge instructions is as important as the actual care they receive. For people who aren't sick enough to be in the ED, the nurse's challenge is to get them into the system and refer them to clinics.

Clinically, there's a difference between urban and suburban trauma. In the suburbs, we don't see as much penetrating trauma (gunshot and stab wounds), but we get a lot more blunt trauma as a result of automobile crashes, homeowner accidents, and sports injuries.

Emergency nursing changes according to the time of day. In general, night patients tend to be sicker, because most people don't want to get out of bed unless it's absolutely necessary. As a result, we have fewer patients at night, but the ones we have are usually worse off.

There are different levels of emergency departments, from the tiny rural department (level four), where patients have to ring the doorbell, to North Shore, which is a level-one trauma center with a helipad and surgeons on call 24 hours a day. Here, we are equipped to handle the most critical patients. For instance, say we are about to receive a 25-year-old male who's been in a serious car crash. He's unconscious, his blood pressure is low, and he has multiple injuries, including fractures of both legs, massive internal bleeding and questionable head trauma. We'll be contacted that the patient is coming, and we will alert the trauma team and prepare the helipad. Before he gets to us, he probably will be intubated. And have multiple IV lines.

When we receive the patient, we take him into the trauma room, which is set up like an OR. While he is being stabilized, two trauma-team nurses will be performing specific, predefined tasks. A third will complete a trauma flow sheet, recording the patient's initial scores and detailing what was done to him before he arrived and what was done after he came in. Typically, we'll have that patient for 15 minutes to an hour, just long enough to stabilize him and send him to surgery if necessary.

That's one end of the spectrum. At the other end, we've established what we call a fast-track emergency service, which is reserved for low-priority patients with minor injuries. This system ensures that such patients don't have to wait hours for service.

Basic decisions in the ED are simple: either admit a patient or treat and release him. Most emergency departments admit between 25 percent and 40 percent of their patients, but some have far higher admission rates. In general, more people are being admitted as our population ages and patients get sicker.

Many patients use the ED to gain access to the hospital, because they can't get in through other channels. And as health care costs rise, emergency departments have become even more oriented to primary care, especially when simple conditions have gone untreated. For example, we see too much pneumonia that progressed from simple cases of flu.

To avoid clogging the emergency department, most hospitals have set up a triage mechanism, in which patients with less-serious conditions are sent to in-hospital clinics. We find that this frees our staff to handle the true emergencies. This is important to the ED nurse, who usually is the patient's first line of defense.

In my department, we work with teams of one physician and three nurses. This means that a nurse is the first professional to see a patient. The nurse takes a history and makes an initial assessment, learning such important details as whether the patient has allergies or is pregnant. For cardiac patients, we take a history, listen to their lungs, and do an EKG. Depending on what we learn from the history and EKG, we may start oxygen and an IV. Traditionally, ED nurses have more responsibility to perform tests and certain technical functions than do floor nurses. But exactly how far that authority extends is very hospital specific.

Of course, a physician must see the patient to make the diagnosis and decision about whether to admit. The outcome hinges on that contact between the nurse and physician, and I find that teamwork between nurses and doctors is stronger in the ED and the OR than in any other hospital departments. On other floors, doctors are in and out, but in emergency they're always present, so the nurses and physicians are able to establish mutual trust.

Emergency department nurses start as floor nurses, but many become certified emergency nurses (CENs) after passing a national certification examination. It's also possible to advance to the level of clinical nurse specialist in emergency, and many ED nurses take courses in trauma, but nothing replaces on-the-job experience. While undergraduate RN programs don't include emergency as a regular rotation, I encourage students to come and check us out. Even for graduate students, emergency department nursing can be very intimidating, and we try to introduce students to the atmosphere of the ED without overwhelming them. While we put them in the middle of the fray, we don't leave them alone, and we never put them in the position of making independent decisions.

Emergency nurses can shape their careers along an administrative track. For example, I have two master's degrees (one in education and one in health care administration), and currently I'm working on my doctorate in nursing administration. I had my initial taste of the administrative side of things in my second job, in which I was head nurse in emergency at a 190-bed community hospital in Long Island. I retained clinical responsibilities, but I also assumed managerial and administrative duties, including drawing up schedules, establishing policies and procedures, and managing a budget. After a year, I went back to the Bronx and became the supervisor of a new emergency department in a 400-bed facility. Construction had just been completed, and I was hired to recruit and train a new staff, establish policies, purchase equipment, and generally elevate the standards of care.

In addition to my current job at the hospital, I'm a faculty member at the Columbia University School of Nursing. In my academic role, I direct the critical care program, teaching critical care and emergency department nursing to 60 graduate students who are working to become clinical nurse specialists. After a year of systems assessment and evaluation, the students spend their second year in a clinical site, assimilating the role of a clinical nurse specialist and completing a project that is intended to synthesize everything they've learned.

In addition, I've established a paramedic training program at the hospital, involving the nurses and physicians. The program covers anatomy, physiology, systems assessment, and initial stabilization, in hopes that we can improve the care patients receive before they reach the hospital. To evaluate patient care, we have a quality-improvement committee made up of nurses, physicians, and prehospital-care providers (eg, EMTs and paramedics). One thing we've done is ensure that every patient with a possible spinal injury comes through the door wearing a cervical collar.

Working in emergency is like living in a fishbowl: It's not easy. It demands great flexibility because you never know what's coming in next. It's extremely stressful, and some nurses have formed informal support groups to let off steam. However, sometimes the strain of juggling 12 or 15 patients can't wait until a weekly group meeting. As a result, the staff can use me as a "sounding board" for those immediate frustrating situations.

The ideal ED nurse must be able to respond to events instantly without allowing the pressure to have an unnerving effect. He — or she — has to be able to balance the euphoria of saving a life against the horrible task of telling a mother her son has died. In spite of this, I've found that once people come to work in emergency, they rarely go anywhere else. In fact, I have never worked in any other area. In emergency, you will be exposed to every specialty — from orthopedics to oncology.

An ED nurse can expect to earn a salary parallel to that in other areas of nursing. Of course, the actual figure depends on the nurse's experience and the cost of living in the area.

To some extent, the pressure of the ED goes unrecognized by other hospital departments because even some of the other head nurses have never set foot in the emergency room. Sometimes, when we're really crowded, I'll bring a head nurse down from one of the other departments and say, "I want you to get an appreciation for this. I want you to know what we're dealing with when we need to transfer a patient upstairs and you tell us the bed isn't ready." Invariably, the reply is, "You're right. I didn't understand."

I think hospital administrators are finally changing their attitude toward emergency departments. Whereas these units used to be considered money-losing but necessary evils, now most emergency rooms are striving to be more consumer oriented. A hospital is a business, and administrators are waking up to the fact that many patients get their first impressions of the hospital from the ED. Increasingly we're being given the equipment we've been clamoring for during the last 10 years. A hospital's front door is not the lobby. It's the emergency department.

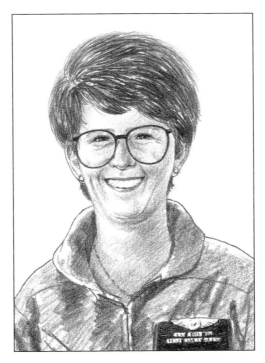

Mary Jo Nimmo, MSN, RN, CNA, EMT,
is program manager of EastCare at
Pitt County Memorial Hospital in
Greenville, North Carolina.

The Flight Trauma Nurse

No doubt about it, being a flight nurse is one of the most exciting practices in nursing today. But is is a very demanding practice that requires the nurse to perform advanced clinical procedures under tremendous pressure and, at times, in extreme conditions. In nearly every case, the patient's life depends on the nurse's abilities. There is no time for second guessing, looking things up, or asking around for opinions. This work is tailor-made for people who can find calm in the midst of chaos. I have been doing this for nine years and I love it.

The basic mission of a flight nurse is to transport critically ill and injured patients from accident scenes or from one medical facility to another. The helicopter we use is actually a mobile intensive care unit that carries virtually all the equipment found in a hospital-based ICU: cardiac and oxygen monitors, blood pressure monitors, defibrillators, intra-aortic balloon pump monitors for heart patients. The only difference is that many of these items have been miniaturized so they will fit in the limited cabin space.

The patients we transport include neonatal and pediatric cases, victims of trauma or cardiac problems, and people who need emergency surgery. The determination of whether to transport a patient by air is made by the physician in charge of the case. In fact, I would like to make it clear that we are acting under a physician's direction at all times. While we serve as the physician's eyes, ears, and hands at the scene and may perform advanced clinical procedures, we do not practice independently. Orders must be issued by a physician for emergency measures more complex than CPR.

We are called to an accident scene for two reasons. The most obvious is that helicopter transport is so fast. We fly faster than 120 miles per hour and we don't have to contend with traffic. We also may be called because we provide a higher level of care than those who might be transporting the patient. This is especially true when multiple drug infusions may be required and the patient's condition is so complicated and volatile that continuity of care must be ensured.

The composition of helicopter crews may vary, depending on a program's mission, area of coverage, and generally accepted local practices. Some fly with a nurse and paramedic, some with a nurse and a physician, and some with a nurse and a respiratory therapist. We fly with two nurses who have received identical training but perform distinctly separate roles. One will be the primary nurse in charge of assessing the patient, discussing the care plan with the physician in charge, and instituting care according to the physician's orders. The secondary nurse is responsible for radio communications, safety in and around the helicopter, loading and unloading equipment, and preparing the patient for transport. This nurse also serves as an extra set of eyes for the pilot. The pilot is not an EMT and, essentially, is restricted to flying the helicopter.

We operate in a 120-mile radius, and nearly 90 percent of the cases we handle are transports between hospitals. For the most part, these involve critical patients who are being transferred to a facility that can provide a more advanced level of care. We can handle as many as six calls a day, but we average two or three. Each takes approximately an hour. Some of my days start at 6:30 AM and don't end until well past 10 at night. In addition to the time we spend flying and caring for patients, we must enter information on the patient's chart, document the physician's orders, keep our own log, and gather various bits of information for our in-house database.

Most programs like this one have a communications center where information is received and relayed to the physician. Once the decision is made to transport, the center pages the flight team and away we go. If we are transporting a patient between hospitals, we are briefed on the history, and we have a good idea of what we will be dealing with. If we are heading to an accident scene, we are facing more unknowns. The best that we can do is get ready and wait to see what we find.

At the scene, we are likely to see multiple injuries, cardiac arrest, and respiratory failure. The care we provide usually depends on how much has been done prior to our arrival. Often, we have to establish an airway and an IV, stabilize the patient on a back board, and apply a cervical immobilization device. Then we "package" the patient for flight — attach the IV lines to pressure bags and make sure no straps or clothing are dangling off the back board — and take off. The IV pressure bags are important because drip-lines are effective only if they are hung high and kept vertical. This is not always possible inside the helicopter's cabin, so the bags ensure a steady flow.

Often we arrive at the scene of an accident and find that the patient has yet to be extricated from wreckage. This happened recently when a log truck crashed head-on into an automobile and then swerved into a creek. The driver was buried in the wreckage under the load of logs, up to his waist in the water. We couldn't see anything but his hand. He was talking, which meant he had an airway, but we didn't know the extent of his injuries. We started an IV of Ringer's solution into his hand because we couldn't even tell if he was bleeding. The only way to free him was to unload the logs one by one. It took two and a half hours before he was out and we could start attending to his injuries. In the meantime, the best we could do was to keep talking to him to keep his spirits up and, hopefully, keep him from passing out. When we finally got to him, we found he had a crushed pelvis but no major organ damage.

While hospital transports are not as exciting as accident scene transports, they are no less serious. We regularly encounter cases of cardiac arrest, respiratory failure, seizures, or multiple organ failure, forcing us to perform advanced emergency procedures. To deal with such situations, flight nurses receive advanced training that is at a higher level than that for hospital-based emergency room or critical care nurses. Techniques we have been certified to perform include cricothyroidotomy, nasal and oral tracheal intubations, needle chest decompression, and placement of femoral and external jugular IV lines.

Even before candidates can be considered for flight nursing, the national standard mandates they have at least two years of critical care experience in a hospital setting. Usually, we look for a little more than that, and most of the applicants we see come from emergency departments and ICU practices.

Our training is individualized so that we train one person at a time. The regimen includes instruction on safety in and around the helicopter, every protocol for the types of patients we see, packaging the patient for flight and the exact duties of the primary and secondary nurses. We tailor the clinical instruction to the needs of each candidate. For instance, if a nurse has a great deal of cardiac experience, we would probably focus more on EMS training. An ED nurse might need more cardiac training. To become familiar with the presentations we see, the candidate must spend time on the units for which we transport: medical, cardiothoracic, surgical, neurologic ICU, and neonatal and pediatric ICU. Once candidates are familiar with protocols and safety techniques, they are paired up with a flight member to begin observing on actual flights. In time, a new nurse will begin functioning as a team member. The entire training process lasts about six weeks. If the candidate is not comfortable by then, or if we don't think she is ready, we will just continue training until she is ready.

The training never really ends, because we are continually learning new procedures and skills. In addition, twice each year we must demonstrate our advanced skills in practice lab sessions.

A flight nurse has to accept the fact that a certain element of danger is associated with this job. We are very conscious of safety at every phase of the flight, but accidents still happen. Several years ago a crew was transporting a critically ill infant. Everything was going normally when suddenly over the radio we heard a crew member say the word *fire*. That was all . . . the radio went blank. The helicopter crashed and everyone on board died. One of the nurses was my best friend and had been in my wedding just three months before. The other nurse was the chief flight nurse, and the pilot was our chief pilot. So along with losing three good friends, we also lost our entire management staff. As a result, I became chief flight nurse and was charged with rebuilding the program.

That was a difficult time for all of us and our families. I remember having a conversation with my husband in which I suggested that maybe I should find a new kind of job. He asked me if I really wanted to do that. I said no. Then he told me that he had always believed there were two kinds of deaths in this world: the kind that comes when your heart stops beating and you die; and the kind you experience when you live to do something, but stop to satisfy others. In the latter case, he believed that you may live on, but it's a living death. My family was very supportive, and so I stayed on. So did all the other staff.

There had been several similar crashes that year, and many hospitals were thinking about suspending their flight services. At the national flight conference I addressed the issue of rebuilding after the crash. I said it would be wrong to suspend our services, because people depend on us to save lives. There are hazards involved, but we recognize them. Nothing in this world is completely safe for anyone, and that's one of the reasons we spend our days rushing patients to hospitals.

It was a pretty passionate speech, and my experience with our own rebuilding gave my opinion a certain credibility. As a result, I was elected to the board of the National Flight Nurses Association. I became involved with strategic planning, and I worked with others to create a certified flight nurse course. I also became involved with the association's safety committee.

Flight nursing is not for everyone because the hours are so long and the tension so high. But to be honest, most of the nurses in this type of practice thrive on stress. The hardest day for most of us to handle is a quiet and uneventful one. However, we work with increments of perfection. After each transport we try to determine whether we could have done anything that would have produced a better outcome. Some people are not comfortable with this sometimes-intense self-criticism, but we think it is essential.

I work with some of the finest nurses in the world. I have a highly autonomous practice and perform advanced procedures. But the best part of my job is being part of a team that saves lives every day. We've had picnics for patients we've helped over the years, and it's incredible to see happy, full-of-life people who were once so close to losing everything. Knowing I had something to do with their survival — well, what could feel better than that?

The Infection Control Nurse

Margaret L. Fracaro, MA (Nursing Administration), RN, CIC, is manager of the infection control program at Columbia Presbyterian Medical Center, New York, New York.

The infection control nurse must be part detective, part diplomat, and part administrator. This specialist also must have strong clinical skills and proven expertise in clinical disease processes, epidemiology, statistics, and the use of computers. Nurses who have this eclectic mix of abilities can look forward to a fascinating practice that is becoming increasingly valued in the hospital and other health care settings.

The enhanced importance of infection control nursing can be attributed to specific facts, chief among which is the impact nosocomial infections have in U.S. hospitals. Each year, over two million patients contract infections while hospitalized; more than 20,000 will die as a direct or indirect result.

AIDS is another reason for the current prominence of infection control. Not only in hospitals, but anywhere there's a chance that health professionals will come in contact with blood or other body fluids, this disease has redefined measures used to prevent infection. Finally, almost every new procedure and advance in medical technology carries the potential for introducing infection and disease. Such advances are taking place at a rapid rate.

Infection control nurses are advocates for patients and staff and provide a service that minimizes the risk of infection and the spread of disease. While many hospitals have physicians and epidemiologists on their infection control teams, I believe nurses are exceptionally well suited to this type of practice. The reason for this lies in the way nurses are educated and in the experience they acquire during clinical practice.

Nurses' education includes courses on pathophysiology, disease processes, and clinical illnesses. Their assessment skills are highly refined, and they are quite knowledgeable about ways in which the clinical environment can impact patients and staff. Most often, it is the staff nurse who carries out the majority of infection control directives.

Infection control is usually organized under a separate department that reports to hospital administration. This liaison is important because administrators are ultimately responsible to the public and regulatory agencies for the quality of patient care. Moreover, they may be liable for negative events. As a result, administrators are usually strong advocates of infection control. They recognize that it is always better to err on the side of caution than to take risks with the health of patients and staff.

In this hospital, the infection control department is staffed by me and the four nurses I supervise. Ours is a multidisciplinary practice in the truest sense of the term: We interact with virtually every department in the hospital. In general, this interaction takes place through surveillance, education, consultations, interventions, or research.

Each of our nurses is assigned to monitor specific areas, and these assignments rotate so the nurses gain familiarity with the entire facility. We usually work regular weekday hours, but emergencies may keep us longer or bring us in on weekends. My staff starts the day by checking to see what happened during the previous 24 hours. Computer programs link us to medical records and to the microbiology lab. Via computer, we are able to perform surveillance on every positive culture in the hospital.

In addition, to make sure the proper precautions are being taken, infection control nurses inspect the units where patients presenting with infectious diseases have been admitted. They see that proper protocols have been followed, and they take steps to make certain that the infection does not spread. If the patient has an infection the unit is not experienced in managing, the infection control nurse provides specialized education and direction for the unit's staff. If the patient presents with a communicable disease that must be reported to the local or state board of health, the infection control nurse handles that responsibility, too.

Educational services are a basic component of infection control. We teach orientation classes on the subject for all new employees, and we offer a more specialized session for physicians and nurses. These classes outline the hospital's infection control program and set forth precautions each employee must follow. For instance, since AIDS began its rampage, universal precautions have become mandatory in all hospitals; we see that health care workers are well versed in those precautions. We also provide in-service presentations that cover special concerns that may be associated with new procedures or equipment. In similar presentations, we detail for staff members the symptoms and potential sources of new types of infections, and we fulfill requirements for information updates as required by such agencies as the Centers for Disease Control and Prevention (CDC), public health departments, or the Joint Commission on Accreditation of Healthcare Organizations (JCAHO). With issues of great concern — say with Legionnaire's disease, toxic shock syndrome, and AIDS — we will provide education as much to allay fears and rumors in the hospital as to inform the staff.

As is true now of tuberculosis, diseases that we thought had been eliminated sometimes reappear. Ten years ago, we saw several cases of TB each year, but these almost always involved patients who had had TB long ago but whose disease was reactivating because their immune systems had weakened. We were not surprised to see two or three new cases each year and as many as two dozen reactivation cases. Today, because of AIDS, homelessness, and other factors, we handle 130 to 140 new cases of TB per year. We find that providing education for staff members helps to insure that TB patients receive appropriate care and also decreases the risk of transmission because personnel understand how to prevent the spread of TB.

Physicians often contact us with questions about how to manage contact after exposure to a particular infectious disease. Nurses call us regarding precautions and procedures used for patients with multiple infections, or to clarify details of isolation. They may want to know what housekeeping procedures should be employed during an infected patient's stay or when normal protocols cannot be followed. We also provide consultation to hospital administrators on such topics as design of patient care areas, interpretation of and adherence to health codes, as well as bed utilization and patient mix. During an outbreak of an infection, or when a patient with a particularly dangerous disease is admitted, our consultations will include details on appropriate precautions, the potential for the infection to spread, and whether such measures as isolating or closing a unit will be necessary. Of course, shutting down a unit or imposing a quarantine is never a popular action. But in some situations, there is no alternative, especially if patients in one unit are contracting the same type of infection and we are unable to isolate its source.

There are also times when a patient presents with a highly infectious disease and a quarantine is instituted to prevent its almost inevitable spread. At times like these, senior staff members of an affected unit may suggest that the infection control department is being overcautious. This is when I must call on all my skills as a diplomat, because we must stand by our findings and not be swayed by less-informed opinions. It is important to remember that our department's decision in such cases may affect the entire hospital. Consequently, we would work with the risk management department to make sure all the necessary documentation is completed and all legal considerations have been weighed.

Our activities even include opportunities for research into new methods of disease prevention and treatment. For example, we recently conducted an investigation into why certain orthopedic patients developed surgical wound infections. The operations were taking place in sterile conditions, and the surgeons followed strict protocols in keeping the area around the wound sterile throughout the procedure. Every precaution had been taken, right down to having the surgical team dress in special spacesuit-type outfits, which turned out to be the problem. The suits allowed the physicians to operate in a relatively germ-free environment but were not being maintained properly. As a result, bacteria were spread to the open wounds through aerosolization. We documented our findings and presented them at a national conference for practitioners in infection control.

Recently, we compared the effectiveness of latex gloves and vinyl ones. There had been a suggestion that gloves made from vinyl were substandard for patient care. However, our study involved more than 100 nurses and showed that the vinyl gloves are just as effective as latex ones. This may not seem like a significant finding until the issue of cost is considered. Vinyl is far less expensive than rubber to produce, and the savings on gloves — omnipresent and disposable in every hospital — were not small at all. These findings were presented at a number of clinical meetings throughout the United States.

A nurse who decides to practice in infection control should have at least three years of clinical practice experience in a hospital. This will give the nurse a solid base of knowledge about disease processes and standard preventive protocols. Clinical experience in ICU, pediatrics, and medicine and surgery provides a particularly good foundation because these areas challenge a nurse's assessment and decision-making skills. Strong communication skills are invaluable as are self-motivation, problem-solving skills, and familiarity with computers.

There is significant autonomy in this field: Nurses are expected to assess a situation and see the possibilities it contains — to think ahead and see "the big picture." Of course, the best way to find out if this career is meant for you is to spend a few shifts with a hospital's infection control team. It also might be wise to look into infection control continuing education offerings. A number of courses offer everything from overviews to intense five-day training.

Should you join an infection control team, you probably will want to earn a master's degree in public health, nursing administration, or some clinical specialty. This is a good credential to have, but it is not immediately essential. After two years of infection control practice, nurses will be eligible to take a certification exam offered by the Association for Practitioners of Infection Control and Epidemiology.

Mine has been an exciting and fascinating career. In all my 20 years in this specialty, I can honestly say that I have continued to learn new things and have been continually challenged by new developments and outbreaks. Every situation offers a different set of clues and a new puzzle to solve. My practice is autonomous and calls on my creativity. I have a great deal of responsibility, but in fulfilling it I have latitude and resources that few other practices could equal. I have worked with virtually every discipline in our hospital and with specialized professionals from the CDC and state and local health departments. I have been able to perform research, publish my findings, and present my work at national forums and conferences. Most important, I believe I have been a direct agent in bringing about changes that significantly improve patient care and the safety of my colleagues.

The Psychiatric Nurse

Mary K. Collins, MS, RN,
is a psychotherapist at the
department of psychiatry at Strong Memorial Hospital,
and an instructor in psychiatric medicine
and health therapy at the University of Rochester
School of Nursing, Rochester, New York.

Much of my time as a psychotherapist is spent helping people cope with distressing situations. I accomplish this directly by working with patients, or indirectly by providing consultation and advice to other therapists. In either case, I believe that my nursing skills give me a distinct advantage over many other practitioners.

Much of what is valuable in psychotherapy comes naturally to nurses. By nature and by training, we tend to be empathetic and nurturing. The specialized education we receive in nursing school gives us the basic medical knowledge necessary to evaluate physical conditions and pharmacokinetic reactions. Our clinical experience has sharpened our assessment, listening, and communication skills. It would be hard to describe a better foundation for a career in this field.

My current practice is split equally between inpatient and outpatient facilities at Strong Memorial Hospital in Rochester, N.Y. The inpatient services I provide are focused entirely on patient care. In our outpatient clinic, I conduct therapy for patients as well as engage in specialized professional consults for other therapists in the Rochester area. Taken together, they make for an ever-challenging practice.

My inpatient practice is located in the psychiatric unit at Strong Memorial and is a collaborative practice with the unit's psychiatrist. We work together as peers coordinating an interdisciplinary team that includes a nurse and a social worker. The unit maintains an average census of seven patients, most of whom present primarily with bipolar disorders.

Bipolar disorders are depressions, the most severe of which is manic-depressive psychosis. Some patients present with symptoms that fit this description exactly. Others are perpetually euphoric, perpetually depressed, or manifest behavior that falls somewhere between the two extremes. When they are in these altered states, patients are much more susceptible to harm. Many become self-destructive or suicidal; others turn their aggressions outward into homicidal activities. I have dealt with both types of patients. Because they are hospitalized, we are able to stabilize their behavior and help them make a transition back to society.

Generally speaking, patients who come into our care follow one of three routes. Some are self-committed and are admitted through our psychiatric emergency room. These individuals may have a history of depression and realize that they need help again. Alternatively, they may be experiencing mental distress for their first time in their life — perhaps extreme depression, repeated suicidal thoughts, or constant agitation. We also have patients whose families or friends called the police to bring them here. Finally, we admit individuals who have overdosed on drugs or attempted suicide. Because of physical complications, these patients will probably spend their first few days on a general medical unit. We admit them after they have recovered sufficiently to begin therapy.

After a patient is admitted, each member of our team has a specific task. The team's physician and I share the responsibility of making mental and physiological assessments and providing therapy. In cases of depression, I immediately try to determine whether the state has been induced by some organic means — say, cocaine or narcotics. If warranted, the patient is checked for brain tumors or other physiological factors that could impair mental health. Because some depression may have a biological foundation, I try to get a complete family history in hopes of finding a possible genetic link. In addition, I attempt to learn whether such environmental stressors as overwork or family strife are an issue. Often, patients who have just been admitted are suffering from severely disrupted sleep patterns. If that is so, I prescribe medication that will help them rest and return to normal sleep habits. It is important to help the patient regain control because altered mental states can pose a danger to the patient and those around him. As a result, I generally prescribe drugs to help stabilize the patient's mood.

Usually it will take two or three days of testing before we can determine the cause of a patient's suffering. During that period we contact the patient's family or friends and gather more data. In most cases, the patient begins to stabilize by this time. This is a critical time in my contact with the patient, because now I lay the foundations for our relationship. If the patient does not see me as someone who can be trusted and can offer help, therapy will be much more difficult. I believe my training as a nurse gives me an advantage at this juncture, because nurses are taught to communicate with patients and to interact with honesty and objectivity. Psychotherapy relies strongly on a practitioners's empathy and ability to listen and understand — all of which are deeply ingrained in nurses. In fact, at this early stage of treatment, just being a nurse to the patient makes a big difference.

Once all members of the team have performed their evaluations and the patient has been stabilized, therapy begins. Therapy will last, on average, between 10 and 21 days and will include private sessions with me or our physician, group sessions, and meetings with a social worker. Patients take part in recreational activities that help them relax and readjust. These activities include woodworking, crafts, physical exercise, and music therapy.

Throughout therapy, it is important for all staff members to be understanding and nonjudgemental. Often, patients have blocked their recollection of behavior that occurred before admission. However, as therapy progresses, memories may begin to surface — perhaps to the patient's embarrassment. For instance, some may have become hypersexual, or they may have run up tremendous credit card bills.

Everything we do is carefully coordinated with team members. We round every day and discuss the progress of each patient. Each week, we meet formally to assess therapy and to discuss plans for care after discharge. The peer relationships among our team members are exceptionally strong. Many nurses are members of multidisciplinary teams, but very few are lucky enough to work in a truly collaborative practice like this one. The autonomy I have enables me to use my skills to their fullest, and this is a significant reward.

While most of our patients are admitted for depression, we also see those with full-blown schizophrenia, victims of incest and rape, and people who display symptoms of posttraumatic stress disorder. Whatever the presentation, our goal is to move the patient out of this setting and back into an outpatient environment. As a result, the plan we devise for each patient's therapy is implemented with an eye toward discharge. We are constantly reevaluating our plan in the light of the patient's progress. This allows us to work with our outpatient facility and other outside resources to make sure all postdischarge services will be available when needed. Depending on the diagnosis, postdischarge care can range from medication and weekly therapy to intensive all-day treatment programs. Most of our patients receive these services at the Mood Disorder Center, our outpatient clinic.

The Mood Disorder Center is a satellite clinic maintained by Strong Memorial's department of psychiatry. Here, I share a collaborative practice with the psychiatrist who is on my inpatient team. My time here is divided between providing therapy for my own patients and offering consultation services for other therapists. The latter is a unique service that we put in place a little over a year ago, when we became aware of the need for support among therapists in the community. Basically, we offer these professionals case evaluations and assessments of psychopharmacotherapy.

Psychopharmacotherapy is a very complex field and, in some ways, finding the right prescription and dosage is almost an art. Many therapists find that what they have prescribed fails to produce the results they intended. In these cases, I review the patient's complete medical and medication history and look for drug interactions or other reasons why the therapy is not producing desired results. My nursing training is advantageous here because I am familiar with pathophysiology and have had intensive instruction on therapeutic agents. To keep these skills fresh, I spend a great deal of time reviewing the current pharmaceutical literature.

We also consult with therapists who have patients that are not progressing on nondrug therapy, so the therapist is looking for advice. In these cases, the therapist forwards the patient's record so I can review the history and the treatments that have been tried thus far. After that, we will have a formal consult in which I offer suggestions for alternate interventions.

In addition to these responsibilities, I see about 20 patients of my own, most of whom present with depression. These people are not as troubled as my inpatients, but many feel they are losing control of their lives. I have them focus on what has been bothering them and then help them develop better skills for coping with the stress that is an unavoidable part of our lives.

All in all, I end up working about 10 to 12 hours a day, five days a week. Beyond that, I share on-call duties with the psychiatrist on my team and must work one weekend each month. Periodically, I also present seminars at the University of Rochester's School of Nursing and am mentor for one student each year.

My professional life is a full one, but it is not without frustrations. For example, my desire to help people is quite strong, and it is difficult to encounter patients I just can't reach. Trying numerous interventions only to realize that the person is not progressing can be extremely disappointing. It becomes even more distressing when my care must be denied for insurance reasons. I don't know how many times I've had to wrestle with an insurance representative who has no knowledge of my patient's history and is second guessing my order for a CAT scan or for a few more days in our facility. Psychiatric care is not like orthopedics or general surgery: recovery is much more difficult to predict. It's frustrating—and frightening, too—to discharge patients before they are ready.

Nurses who are interested in a career as a therapist should first gain one or two years of clinical experience in general nursing, because physiological assessment and bedside care skills are essential. Moreover, I recommend spending time observing a hospital's inpatient psychiatric unit and talking with nurses and therapists there about their activities. It may also be useful to get the perceptions of a therapist in private practice. At a minimum, it is necessary to have a master's degree in nursing and to become certified as a therapist.

Few professions offer the flexibility of nursing. Nurses need to take advantage of that flexibility and shape their practices into a form that nurtures their aspirations and interest while providing the opportunity for professional and personal growth. For me, psychotherapy has been a perfect fit.

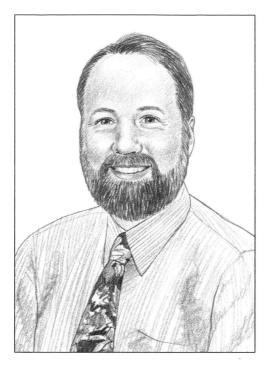

*Larry Scahill, MSN, MPH, RN,
is a clinical nurse specialist and
associate research scientist at the
Child Study Center at the Yale University
School of Medicine,
New Haven, Connecticut.*

The Child Psychiatric Nurse

Although nursing is commonly recognized as one of the oldest health care professions, formal training is relatively new. Specialty practice, in which the nurse acquires advanced training in a specific clinical area, is even newer. Indeed, most contemporary nursing specialties, including psychiatry, primary care, emergency care, and oncology, have emerged since World War II. Perhaps the most visible of these is the nurse practitioner specialty, which came on the scene in the mid-1960s.

Nurses choose their specialties in a variety of ways. For some, work experience in a particular field prior to nursing school is the determinant. Others develop an interest in a specialty after completing basic nursing education and working as a staff nurse in that field. In either case, graduate study is now regarded as a prerequisite for advanced practice in a clinical specialty of nursing.

I began working in the mental health field soon after graduating from high school in the late 1960s. At the time, I was working in an urban community center that provided free meals and clothing to the homeless and inner-city poor. This was an era of great changes in psychiatry. The advent of psychopharmacologic drugs brought new hope and understanding to the major mental illnesses. The large state hospitals were rapidly reducing their patient populations in a policy called deinstitutionalization. I witnessed the dramatic effect of this policy on the urban landscape as many of these chronically ill individuals wound up homeless and on the streets. After four years of working in the urban center, I entered nursing school with a keen interest in psychiatry.

In the late 1970s, upon completion of my undergraduate training, I accepted a position in a community mental health center that served a rural population and provided services to individuals and families of all ages. It was in this setting that I started doing clinical work with children. Although I had no specific training in child psychiatry at the time, there were few psychiatric clinicians in this rural community. Thus, in large measure, my initiation to child psychiatry was prompted by institutional necessity.

A few years later, I took a job as a staff nurse in a leading child psychiatric hospital on the East Coast. There I had the opportunity to work with expert child psychiatric clinicians and researchers, and this heightened my interest in child psychiatry and sparked an interest in research.

Compared with other health professions, nursing is unusual in that a person can work at a basic level in a specialty area after graduation. Moreover, it is clear that staff nurses in such fields as cardiology, oncology, or child psychiatry often develop solid clinical skills without graduate training. However, graduate education fosters greater expertise in a chosen clinical specialty and assures greater independence in practice. In my own case, I worked for about six years in child psychiatry before entering a graduate training program.

There are approximately 12 graduate programs for child and adolescent psychiatric nursing in the United States. These programs usually last three to four semesters. All require applicants to have a bachelor's degree and most, but not all, require that the degree be in nursing. There are a few programs that combine basic nursing education with specialty training and admit nonnurse college graduates. These programs usually require six to eight semesters of study.

To pursue my interests in clinical child psychiatry and research, I entered a joint graduate program in child psychiatric nursing and public health. This is a three-year, dual-degree program that leads to two master's degrees. Upon graduation, I joined the faculty of the Child Study Center in the School of Medicine at Yale University. More recently, I have been appointed to the clinical faculty of the Yale University School of Nursing.

In my current position, I have administrative, clinical, and research responsibilities in the tic disorder and obsessive-compulsive disorder clinics. These clinics provide evaluation and treatment for children with tic disorders and obsessive-compulsive disorders and are the center of an active research program.

Tic disorders are characterized by involuntary movements and vocalizations. Motor tics often include eye blinking, facial grimacing, and shoulder shrugging. Vocal tics typically consist of repetitive throat clearing, grunting, and repeating syllables or words. Motor and vocal tics may be transient or chronic and may occur separately or together. When both motor and vocal tics persist, the disorder is termed *Tourette's syndrome* (TS).

Obsessive-compulsive disorder (OCD) is defined by the presence of recurring thoughts (obsessions) and ritualized behaviors (compulsions). Until recently, OCD was considered rare in adults and even less common in children. However, recent data indicate that it is not so uncommon, and studies from specialty clinics, including our own, confirm that the disorder can be fully expressed in children.

Both Tourette's syndrome and OCD have their onset in childhood, and both tend to be chronic. They are often called neuropsychiatric disorders because of the accumulating evidence that supports a neurobiological basis for these disorders. There has been an increased interest in the disorders in recent years because, in addition to the fact that they are more common than previously believed, they provide models for exploring the interaction of genetic endowment and environment in the elaboration of a clinical syndrome. Effective treatment demands an appreciation of the biological underpinnings of these disorders as well as a recognition of their psychological and social implications.

As a child psychiatric nurse practitioner in this setting, I provide direct clinical services as an independent clinician and as a member of a multidisciplinary team. Referrals to the clinic, approximately three per week, come from a variety of sources including child psychiatrists, neurologists, pediatricians, psychologists, clinical nurse specialists, and school personnel. New cases are evaluated by a team consisting of a child psychiatrist and a child psychiatric nurse specialist. The evaluation entails a review of standardized rating scales and questionnaires; a careful survey of the onset and progression of primary symptoms; an assessment of past medical, developmental, psychiatric, and family histories; and a review of prior treatment.

Follow-up care is also a collaborative effort. Despite growing evidence that TS and OCD are neurobiological disorders, treatment is not solely pharmacologic. Some children with TS may need pharmacologic treatment for tics, while others may need intervention for associated behavior problems, such as inattention, overactivity, and impulsiveness. For still others, psychotherapy is indicated to ensure optimal adjustment in the face of a chronic condition. In addition, education for the family and the school often is required in order to foster an understanding of the involuntary nature of tics and of the importance of providing structure and setting limits on the child's impulsive behavior. Finally, if a child is treated with medication, the referring clinician, school personnel, and parents need to know the purpose, side effects, and dose of the medication. The availability of the child psychiatrist or the child psychiatric nurse practitioner ensures better access to families, outside clinicians, and school personnel.

This model of multidisciplinary teamwork applies equally well to the treatment of childhood OCD. I am often involved in educating parents, pediatricians, mental health professionals, and school personnel about the disease. For example, in their efforts to help the child, many parents inadvertently participate in the child's rituals. When this occurs, it usually happens gradually, and parents often need guidance about how to avoid further participation. Also, because the medications used to treat OCD are relatively new, requests for information about their use and side effects are commonplace.

The range of research projects devoted to TS and OCD is extremely wide and includes both the treatment and causes of these disorders. These research activities are conducted by a multidisciplinary group that includes geneticists, neuroanatomists, neurochemists, physicians, psychologists, and psychiatric nurse practitioners. I participate in the design of research projects. I also recruit subjects, perform clinical assessments of these subjects, and often take part in the analysis of data (statistics was a central part of my training in public health).

Some of the research projects, such as the search for the gene that causes TS, are being conducted in collaboration with other institutions. I am not involved in the laboratory work concerning the genetics of Tourette's syndrome. But I do take part in group discussion about the status of this research effort and its relevance to patient care.

In contrast, I am very involved in the multicenter treatment trial of a new drug for the treatment of children with OCD. I coordinate the screening and entry into the study and serve as the primary clinician for children in the study. Multicenter trials such as this one are likely to be more common in the future and will have considerable impact on clinical care.

Another current project uses magnetic resonance imaging (MRI) to measure the three-dimensional volume of specific brain structures that may be relevant to the pathophysiology of TS and OCD. Of particular interest in this study are the basal ganglia, which have been implicated in movement disorders and OCD.

I also coordinate clinical services in the tic disorder and OCD clinics. This involves managing the operation of the clinic, screening and scheduling new patients, oversight of billing, ensuring the quality and confidentiality of patients' records, maintaining clinic supplies, and supervising clinic personnel.

Psychiatry is in an era of tremendous change. Accumulating findings from genetics, neuroimaging, and neuropsychopharmacology provide compelling evidence in favor of neurobiological origins for many of the major psychiatric disorders. The proliferation of psychopharmacologic agents holds promise for better treatments of psychiatric disorders but will demand a higher level of expertise for all nurses working in psychiatry and for psychiatric nurse practitioners in particular — especially as more states grant prescriptive authority to nurses in advanced practice roles. Accordingly, graduate school programs in child psychiatric nursing will undoubtedly include more neurobiology and psychopharmacology.

Efforts to contain health care costs will undoubtedly place more stringent limits on hospital stays and the number of outpatient visits. On the other hand, health care reform promises better access to mental health treatment for those who are currently uninsured. The resulting increased demand for mental health services offers an exciting opportunity for child psychiatric nurse practitioners. To make the most of this opportunity child psychiatric nurse practitioners will need to articulate clearly the nature and scope of their practice to the public, to other professionals, and to policy makers.

In short, child psychiatric nursing is in a time of great challenge and opportunity. Nurses with advanced training are poised to expand the scope of their clinical practices and to achieve even greater independence. They also will be able to find greater opportunities in clinical research and health policy.

Specialty practice in child psychiatric nursing is a thriving profession with a national organization with chapters across the country, a peer-review journal, and professional certification through the American Nurses Association. Preparation for independent practice in child psychiatric nursing requires graduate education at least at the master's level. In the future, child psychiatric nursing will be more biological in its orientation, although psychological and social concerns will not be neglected. The basic sciences, genetics, and pharmacology will become increasingly important to clinical practice. Few areas of nursing offer this variety, this independence, or these rewards.

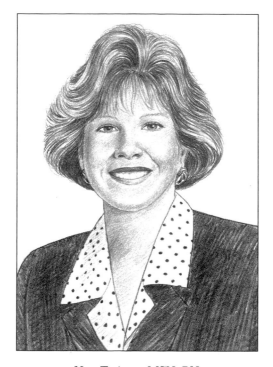

Nan Troiano, MSN, RN,
is an associate in obstetrics and gynecology,
and codirector of critical care obstetrics at
Vanderbilt University School of Medicine,
Nashville, Tennessee.
She also is president of
Harvey, Troiano & Associates, Inc., and a
consultant in private practice in
Houston, Texas.

The Perinatal Nurse Specialist

I didn't want everything from my nursing career, just variety, independence, an advanced clinical practice, and the chance to collaborate with other health care providers. And I wanted all of this on my own terms. I found all of these elements as I carved out my own specialty as a perinatal nurse specializing in critical care obstetrics. In this role I work exclusively with women who have high-risk pregnancies, providing primary care as well as intensive care should they require hospitalization. I also teach students and hospital staff about critical care obstetrics.

But I was skeptical when my college counselor suggested I consider nursing. I pictured myself as a career nonconformist, and my impression of nurses didn't fit. I thought of nurses as women who wore white hats and white hose and worked limited roles reporting to physicians. A few conversations with practicing nurses changed my mind. Two avenues in particular appealed to me. The first was working as a nurse midwife in a low-risk, health-oriented career. The second was nursing in acute care settings, which encompassed a collaborative practice with physicians and required a strong knowledge base in applied science.

After two years at the Tuscaloosa campus of the University of Alabama, I transferred to Huntsville to finish a four-year nursing degree. When it came time to apply for a job and choose a specialty, I was torn between obstetrics and critical care. Finally, I requested the ICU or ER. Then fate stepped in—there were no openings in critical care settings, but there was one in labor and delivery. I took the job and loved it. Nevertheless, my affinity for intensive care kept surfacing as I found myself gravitating to the sickest patients. I wanted to blend the wonder of childbirth with the challenge of managing complications.

I spent five years at Huntsville Hospital, first as a staff nurse and then as a charge nurse. I firmly believe that all nurses need to test the theoretical principles they learn in school in the reality of the hospital setting. One discrepancy was immediately apparent to me. I noticed that many competent nurses, particularly those who had come from AD programs, seemed to feel uncomfortable working with highly scientific information. They appeared not to understand the physiological principles underlying some routine procedures.

Fetal monitoring, for instance, was available in many nonacademic settings only after 1980. So, suddenly, personnel who had been schooled before this time found themselves grappling with equipment that provided information about a baby's heart rate and a mother's patterns of uterine activity. Some found it very difficult to understand. While the mechanics of the machine had been explained, the basis for the information it provided was not. Consequently, fetal monitoring was regarded as just another procedure, which is an attitude that relegates nurses to a task-oriented role. I was sufficiently concerned about this situation that I was asked to teach in-service courses on the physiology behind various fetal heart rate patterns.

Teaching came naturally for me, and in my third year I took a position in perinatal outreach, where I worked with obstetrics nurses and physicians in 21 outlying hospitals. Those rural facilities often dealt with complicated pregnancies among women who had limited access to prenatal care or who faced adverse social situations. By my fourth year I knew that if I wanted to continue teaching and command my ideal job, I needed better credentials.

I entered graduate school at Vanderbilt University, working for the School of Medicine as an outreach coordinator. Again, I taught nurses and helped them gain practical experience in our hospital. During this time my academic adviser became my mentor. Professionally, she was doing everything I wanted to do. She had even taken what seemed to me the ultimate step of entering into joint practice with a physician. Seeing a nurse and physician work as colleagues without an underlying "us versus them" attitude was liberating.

When I finished graduate school in 1987, obtaining a master's in parent-child nursing, I accepted a faculty appointment at Vanderbilt's medical school as an associate in obstetrics and gynecology. I teach various aspects of high-risk obstetrics to medical students, both before and after an obstetric rotation. However, I mostly work with and teach critical care obstetrics to OB/GYN residents and fellows in maternal-fetal medicine. I'm aware of few other places where nurses have such an opportunity. Because I also have hospital privileges, I'm able to work with, teach, and support the nursing staff in the obstetric ICU. I also teach in the school of nursing as the director of the graduate program in OB critical care.

By 1988, I realized that the population of obstetric patients had become increasingly complex in the decade since I entered OB nursing. There were more women becoming pregnant who had significant chronic medical illnesses, such as heart disease, pulmonary complications, and serious hypertension. In many of the areas we served, there was little or no prenatal care. There were drug problems, battered and abused women, and environmental stressors. On top of all that, there were the general stresses of modern life.

These factors produced complicated pregnancies as well as disjointed health care. For instance, a pregnant woman with heart disease was likely to be referred to a cardiologist, because the obstetrics department was uncomfortable with cardiac disease. The cardiologist was equally unfamiliar with pregnancy and would treat the patient as a woman with heart disease, not a pregnant woman with heart disease. Women were being treated in bits and pieces, and I knew that had to change.

In 1987, I began to collaborate with another clinical nurse specialist, and we forged an important relationship with a perinatologist who was conducting clinical research in critical care obstetrics. He said he had never worked with obstetrics nurses like us, who had solid physiological training and were interested in patient research. His research required data collection and delivery of sophisticated patient care around the clock. He recognized that development of a specialty nursing practice in this area would facilitate the continued growth of the specialty, and we committed to working together toward this goal. Collaborating with him was a crucial step in establishing the specialty as a recognized discipline. Nationally, only a handful of nurses were working in this field. And even though we knew one another, we needed access to the medical information that was being gathered in this highly specialized area. Nurses and physicians have distinct knowledge bases, but there is significant overlap in critical care.

The fact that I had gained expertise in such a new specialty led to an interesting business opportunity. A nurse colleague and I started a consulting business in which we design OB intensive care units and provide educational support for physicians and nurses. In addition, we developed a national conference for nurses on critical care obstetrics, which we hold several times a year. In general, we enroll only experienced obstetrics nurses, and expose them to advanced concepts in critical care. The course work centers on case studies that we use to introduce procedures such as invasive hemodynamic monitoring or mechanical ventilation, as well as disease processes that might complicate pregnancy.

While I travel on business several days a month, I spend most of my time in the university hospital, clinic, or classroom. Clinic work occupies approximately two days a week in a joint practice I and two other clinical nurse specialists share with a perinatologist. We provide complete prenatal care for patients who have high-risk pregnancies, or who have the potential for developing complications. If we treat patients in the early stages of pregnancy, it is easier to manage them if they must be admitted to the ICU later.

Often, there is a rigid division of functions between an obstetrician and an obstetrics nurse. The nurse gathers assessment data to present to the physician, who interprets it and plans care. In my role as an advanced practice nurse in critical care OB, I provide prenatal care to high-risk pregnant women. This may include performing the initial history and physical exam, taking a Pap smear, and providing prenatal counseling. Throughout her pregnancy I collaborate to reevaluate the woman's risk status, order surveillance tests, and interpret results. Not only does this give me a larger practice role, but it also facilitates continuity in patient care.

All too often, an obstetrician's practice is structured so that a patient may spend as little as 15 minutes with the doctor during each office visit. In many cases, this leaves large gaps in the patient's prenatal education and understanding of the plan of care. In my practice, patients have more time allotted for education. When medical interventions are necessary, collaboration with the perinatologist is sought. Working together, we are able to promote more consistent, quality care.

The time I spend at the outpatient clinic dovetails with the four to five days a week I'm on 24-hour call for the hospital's OB-ICU unit, of which I am codirector. We have a staff of 22 and treat an average of one critical care patient a week (average stay: 72 hours). By introducing critical care in an obstetric setting, pregnancy remains the focus of a woman's condition. Because we have often been the provider of the patient's prenatal care, we know the patient better than a medical ICU staff would.

This approach is highly beneficial from a clinical standpoint, as well as from a psychosocial one. Even the sickest of patients envisions herself surrounded by her family as she delivers a normal, healthy baby. Unfortunately, adult visitors are often limited in regular ICUs, and bringing a baby or other siblings in would be out of the question. But maternity is the focus in our ICU. We often have patients who are dependent on a ventilator and have invasive hemodynamic monitoring devices in place, but we try to treat the unit just like any other labor and delivery room: We fill it with flowers and stuffed animals, and we bring the baby in to stay as its condition permits. We even set up beds so the patient's family can sleep in the same room with the patient.

I make rounds with the attending perinatologist and the chief resident in the OB-ICU unit, discussing the status and treatment of patients. For instance, I may recommend ventilator changes and interpret hemodynamic and oxygen transport data in order to plan pharmacologic intervention. In a traditional labor and delivery unit, I may not be able to have this level of involvement. But here, I've developed a rapport with the attending perinatologists, and they feel free to ask for my opinion. They know what I feel comfortable with, and they trust me. In some instances, the perinatologist has asked me to admit a patient, perform the initial work-up, develop admission orders, then review it with the residents. Physicians have the final authority, but they give me latitude to operate autonomously.

While I relish the opportunity to write my own job description, I think it's unwise to jump into a nontraditional role before establishing a firm foundation in clinical practice. Often this experience must be gained in a traditional setting. Nurses in our critical care OB unit must have three years' staff nursing experience in labor and delivery in a tertiary care teaching hospital, where they will have worked with high-risk obstetric patients.

Within my specialty, perinatal nursing with critical care obstetrics, there are other ways to carve out a career. Certainly teaching is an option. Consulting is another, especially concentrating on hospital staff development. Or a perinatal nurse could choose to work with low-risk, normal pregnancies, becoming a nurse practitioner and providing primary health care, then referring the patient to a physician for delivery.

Organized OB-ICU care is still rather rare, and few units exist outside of a teaching hospital. In fact, the most frustrating thing about my career is that OB critical care is so new that I sometimes feel somewhat isolated.

My greatest professional rewards lie in seeing the system work for patients. In one case, an Amish woman in her 13th pregnancy began hemorrhaging and was brought to us by helicopter. You can imagine the shock of her relatives, who were as unfamiliar with hospitals as they were with helicopters. It was clear that we had not only her physical care to consider, but also the emotional care of her family. Her bleeding was so profuse that she was admitted to the OB-ICU requiring invasive hemodynamic monitoring and mechanical ventilation prior to a hysterectomy after the delivery. As soon as she was stable, we turned our attention to her family. We brought them into the unit, where they sang lullabies to the new baby. When the mother awoke from sedation, she wrote a note asking to see her baby, and soon she was breast feeding. Surrounding this patient with a familiar social context was extremely important, but it couldn't have been done without the clinical resources to back it up. At one point during this patient's recovery a resident walked in and said, "You have a woman on a ventilator breast feeding a baby. Now I've seen everything." Granted, that may seem a bit unorthodox. But when I asked him how he felt about it, he said, "If my wife had trouble with a pregnancy, this is where I would want her to be."

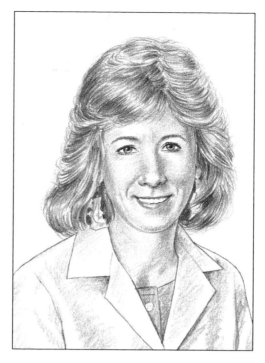

Ria Hawks, MS, RN, OCN,
is a research nurse clinician at
the Babies & Children's Hospital of New York,
Columbia Presbyterian Medical Center,
and an associate on the special instructional
faculty at Columbia University
School of Nursing,
New York, New York.

The Pediatrics Inpatient Nurse

Every day I relive my childhood. I wear animal earrings, play games, and make calendars with stickers on them. My world may be a child's world, but it's not all fun and games: I practice in the division of pediatric hematology/oncology.

Once I worked in politics and later in costuming, and those activities sometimes made me the center of attention at cocktail parties. But when I changed careers, I quickly learned that the words *pediatric oncology* have a dampening effect on conversation. People think I must have an inherently depressing job, but it's not.

In 1970, I graduated from college with a degree in history. Although the world of the theatre was exotic, the spirit of the 1960s emerged, and I longed for a more meaningful career. A couple of years later I enrolled in a two-year BSN program for college graduates at Columbia University's School of Nursing. I put myself through school by working as an aide in pediatrics and fell in love with it. Not only did I like the kids, I enjoyed the environment, and I felt that pediatrics nurses had good rapport with physicians.

I graduated in 1974 and went to work as a staff and charge nurse. Then from 1976 to 1982 I was head nurse of a 15-bed pediatric neurology unit. After a brief stint in administration, I decided my talents and interests lay in clinical applications, and in 1983 I came to Babies & Children's Hospital at Columbia Presbyterian. I've been here for the last 10 years.

Although this division follows a large number of hematology patients, I work strictly in oncology, almost exclusively with inpatients — about 15 at any one time. My job involves patient care, but my duties are varied, including consultation, research, and teaching. Although I am a research nurse clinician, my duties closely resemble those of an advanced practice clinical nurse specialist. In fact, I recently received a master's as clinical nurse specialist in pediatric oncology.

My day-to-day duties include coordinating chemotherapy, admissions, and supportive care for our pediatric oncology and bone marrow transplant patients. I supervise the care delivered by staff nurses, and I am accountable for the quality of nursing care on the inpatient unit. Moreover, I coordinate the nursing plans for complex therapies. And because I understand treatment protocols and rationales as well as the potential for drug toxicity, I'm well qualified to communicate knowledge on these subjects to the house medical staff and to set parameters for the nursing staff. For example, I often assist physicians in writing orders. They may know what drugs should be used, but they may not understand the details of administering the agents. But I do know the mechanics of IVs and can suggest ways to solve most problems that arise with this route of administration. I can discuss therapies with the attending physician and interpret the orders for interns and the nursing staff. While the physician chooses drugs and determines dosages, it is not uncommon for me to be asked to take part in decision making.

In larger hospitals, a team of chemotherapy nurses is responsible for giving intravenous push chemotherapy. In our relatively small unit, the job falls to me. Interns are authorized to perform this procedure, but I know the patients and am better able to find veins and use IV lines. Infusional chemotherapy is hung by a staff nurse, and my role is to identify potential problems and make recommendations when problems arise. I'm a source of information for our nurses, and I coordinate the care of our patients with other hospital departments, such as physical therapy or psychology.

I make rounds in the morning, making pretreatment evaluations of children admitted the night before. If I find problems, I discuss them with the staff. If I can't solve a problem, I find someone who can. I confirm the day's schedule, review admission orders, and work with families to educate them about aspects of the care their children are receiving. In the case of a child whose cancer has just been diagnosed, I meet with the parents to review the disease process and to tell them what they might expect within the next several weeks. We talk about chemotherapy and its possible side effects. I give them a calendar that tells them when the child will come to the hospital, and I outline what they might look for during the month. For instance, within a week to 10 days after chemotherapy, the child will be at greatest risk for infection. Consequently, I note that the parents should be especially alert and careful during that period.

Much of my work has to do with the psychology of children and their families. I assess the dynamics of each family, including the emotional state of both child and parents as well as available support systems. I worry about the family's ability to afford treatment and to provide the care that will be necessary at home. If there are problems, I try to find resources to solve them. Relying on the information I gather, I work with the physician and, frequently, a psychologist or social worker in developing discharge plans.

In one case, the little girl's mother was a nurse and thoroughly competent to do whatever procedures were necessary at home. However, the mother confided to me that this was too much for her, partly because her husband didn't feel capable of helping. To solve these problems, I organized sessions in which the father became involved and learned to do some of the work himself thereby relieving the mother from carrying all the responsibility. We also enlisted the grandmother's help. In the end, we were able to decrease the mother's work load and anxiety while accommodating the child's desire to be treated at home.

Usually, the longer a child is sick, the more the family values the child's time at home and the more skilled they become at providing the necessary care. Obviously, a family that has to deal with cancer must endure a terrible amount of anxiety and anger. It is not unusual for some of that anger to be aimed at the staff who care for the child. In my job, I identify the problem and work with the therapist and social worker to redirect the anger and help the patient deal with the stress of living with cancer.

A significant part of my job is organizational, doing paperwork or making sure admission beds are ready on time. I follow up on the results of blood tests and take care of discharges. I make sure that nurses and physicians have updated summaries of information so that they're aware of recent admissions and why those new patients have been admitted: Is it time for a chemotherapy treatment? Does the patient have an infection?

To succeed in this practice, a nurse must be clinically skilled and well organized, as well as flexible enough to adapt if things don't go according to plan. Caring for children requires patience, creativity, and keen observational skills. Providing nursing care for the child with cancer also involves caring for the family as a whole.

No family is ever the same after cancer has been diagnosed. It changes a family's value system along with its hopes and dreams. A staff nurse cares for a patient and his family through teaching as well as delivering nursing care. As a clinical nurse specialist, I instruct the family about which toxicities to anticipate and what the medical staff can do to prevent or minimize them. More important, I teach the family members what they can do themselves to lessen the side effects, feel better, and return to as normal a life as possible. I assist the families in setting goals — short-term as well as long-term ones — and try to reduce the impact the disease will have on their lives.

My job has evolved over the decade from one of patient care to one that requires me to coordinate and direct the efforts of others. For instance, I now do more formal staff teaching, as well as arranging for discharge and home care. And as advanced technology enters the home care environment, my job is shifting in that direction. For instance, when I first started working with cancer patients, it was beyond imagination that chemotherapy could be given at home. Today, I coordinate home care that includes chemotherapy, and I am on call for parents who need help.

Beyond my clinical responsibilities, I serve as a consultant to hospital administrators. For example, at a recent meeting on reimbursement procedures for chemotherapy and bone marrow transplants, I was the expert who outlined specifically what is involved in the procedures and identified the areas that should be charged to generate revenue. In cases where specialized, one-on-one care is needed, I'm expected to justify that need.

One of our main responsibilities in pediatric oncology nursing is to help the children we care for understand what's happening to them so they can learn to cope with their fears and anxieties. We encourage them to participate in the struggle to get better. If we can ease their suffering and help them gain some control over their lives, we free them to get on with the business of childhood. That's important work.

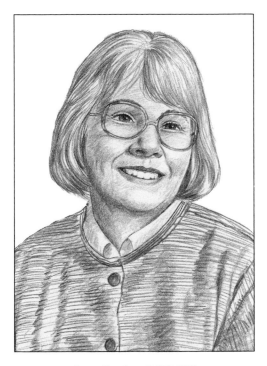

*June Conlon, BSN, RN,
is a school nurse at
Pleasantville Middle School,
Pleasantville, New York.*

The School Nurse

Nursing in a school allowed my schedule to coincide with that of my children. This meant I would always be home when they needed me. Combined with my sixth sense for kids, that made a school a perfect practice site for me.

The school nurse can choose among a wide diversity of options. Positions are available in urban, suburban, or rural settings at elementary, middle school, or high school levels. I spent my first 15 years in the same suburban high school my children attended. I liked the high school age group, and I felt comfortable with the family structures common to this group. Two years ago I was transferred to the middle school.

Taking care of children's physical needs, keeping height and weight charts, and performing eye and ear tests are only a fraction of the school nurse's job. These tasks are not the total focus of school nursing. In a high school, clinical responsibilities often are negligible. Indeed, most of the students I saw were seeking emotional aid, support, or direction. Real medical emergencies were rare, although I needed the skills to deal with them when they occurred.

Many children are reluctant to talk to their parents about problems, so the nurse often is their first recourse. Because the emotional pressures on a high school student can be very intense, I spent a great deal of time talking to young people about aspects of their home and family life., and frequently I felt like a surrogate mother.

Here at the middle school, parents still keep close watch over their children. However, at the high school, children are more inclined to seek out someone other than a parent. As a result, the high school students often seemed to be extensions of my own family, especially when they had problems I had experienced with my children. I didn't hesitate to share my personal life with them if I thought it would help them to open up and share their problems. For example, if a student was having a problem with drug abuse, I could relate details of my son's similar experience. If a child's parents were getting divorced, I could talk about my divorce and its effects on my children.

The school nurse must make some tricky judgement calls in the area of confidentiality and legal responsibility. For instance, if I discovered that a child was being physically abused at home, I was obligated to report it to the proper authorities. When there were reports that a child was being abused, it would be my job to confirm this. Absolute judgment calls are difficult because it sometimes is necessary to preserve a gray area of protection for yourself. For instance, if I smell alcohol on a student's breath, he can easily deny that he has been drinking. If the parents take his side, it all boils down to my word against his.

If a school nurse learns that a student has tried to commit suicide, or is talking about doing so, the nurse has no choice but to report it. On the other hand, if a girl wants information about Planned Parenthood, or confesses that she thinks she is pregnant, the nurse could be helpful. My responsibility here is crystal clear, and I simply do my best to make the student understand that it's important to get help. While school nurses may not teach sex education in a formal way, kids often come to ask questions. In such cases, it's important not to make assumptions about their sexual activity. Instead, I wait until they broach the subject. Many conversations with teenagers are of a confidential nature, and in such circumstances a school nurse is very vulnerable and thus has to make sound judgement calls.

The emotional problems young people face often manifest themselves in physical symptoms. While there always will be children who fake a headache or stomachache in order to miss a test, more often than not the complaint is real. A school nurse tries to figure out why. Has the child's mother recently been admitted to the hospital? Are there problems at home? I usually was able to get high school students to sit down and talk about whatever was bothering them. It's somewhat harder to do this with younger children who do not realize that their physical problems can be rooted in psychological distress. With these students, I explain that all people do things that signal they are upset. Some people bite their fingernails, others twirl their hair, and some people get headaches. When children start to understand that there may be an underlying reason for their physical problems, the possibility that the nurse or someone else can help them increases significantly.

Most school nurses without graduate education and certification are strictly limited when it comes to treatment. For example, they cannot give any medications, although certified PNP's do have authority in some schools to prescribe medications. It's frustrating not to be able to deal with simple, obvious problems because there is only so much the school nurse can legally do. I transfer the responsibility back to the parents who frequently take the child home or come to school and administer a medication (eg, Tylenol® for headache) themselves. Because I'm in a small community, I have a relationship with the parents of many of my kids, so it's easy for me to say, "Let's call your mother."

Parental attitudes and family structures have changed a great deal since my arrival 25 years ago. The economy also has changed, so that now almost all mothers work, and they often send their children to school even when they know they are ill. In times past, almost all kids came from traditional, two-parent families. Now, divorce is so widespread that fully a third of students live in single-parent families. Children's behavior has changed too. For example, 20 years ago students vented their frustrations by breaking windows. Today, they are more likely to turn to drugs and alcohol.

I am distressed by the home situations of many of my students, but I'm constantly amazed at their ability to survive. I have a fifth-grade girl who was adopted. Although the parents are divorcing, the father still lives in the house — a situation that can definitely affect the child. While in school she got her first menstrual period, and her mother confessed to me that she'd been dreading this day. When the child came into my office crying and fearful, it fell to me to say, "How wonderful, honey! Welcome to the woman's world."

School nurses need to maintain sharp skills in first aid, they must be able (under doctor's orders) to administer insulin to a diabetic, and they must handle crowd control is someone has an epileptic seizure. They must also know when it's time to declare an emergency and call an ambulance. One school nurse literally had an epidemic on her hands as a result of contaminated cafeteria food. She had to call in emergency services and triage dozens of sick children.

When I became a school nurse, I believe my experience with children was the best thing I could have had on my resume. In terms of formal training, I graduated with a BSN in the late 1940s. I worked in institutional nursing and in social work for a couple of years before I married. I worked weekends in hospitals while I raised my children. Today, a good candidate for school nursing would have a BSN with background in public health nursing and knowledge and experience with children. Few school districts require credentials beyond an RN. In truth, I think a suitable personality is more important than an advanced education in this practice. The effective school nurse must be responsive to children and families and have insight into the effects today's society is having on both. Careful planning is a significant part of the nurse's responsibility, but she must be flexible enough to discard the plan as soon as the day threatens to get out of hand.

In many school districts, including mine, nurses are responsible for tracking attendance. Often they know which children are home ill and which have left the building — as well as where they went and why. In addition, when children return to school after an illness, they may be screened by the nurse to make sure they're well enough to be back. On a typical day, it might take me all morning to get through attendance chores. If the parents are conscientious about calling in, I have less work to do, but it's important to connect with them in some way. Meanwhile, I'm being interrupted by students who need my attention. Someone once said that if a school nurse ever complains of boredom, she's not doing her job. That is very true.

Even though the settings school nurses work in, and the responsibilities they have are very individual, they have many issues in common. As a result, the School Nurses Association — a national organization — was started about five years ago to establish guidelines for different aspects of school nursing and to discuss issues that may affect us all. For example, most of us are seeing increased incidence of child and drug abuse and less parental contact. In many urban areas, we're beginning to see the second generation of AIDS children. I see many asthmatic children in my district.

I should mention that while a school nurse's responsibility revolves mainly around students, there is interaction with the faculty. Even though I'm not in a strict clinical setting, many feel comfortable enough to ask me to take their blood pressure or to talk to me about their own medical conditions.

A school nurse is part counselor, part clinician, and part troubleshooter. Her duties have to do with many aspects of a child's life. Unfortunately, the salaries school nurses receive do not reflect the value or responsibilities of their job. For most, school nursing usually provides a supplementary income. Nevertheless, it is not a supplementary job, because working with children is a demanding and fatiguing occupation. Still, the issue of income fades when I realize how much these students need their school nurse. It's fulfilling to be in the supermarket and hear a child say, "Hey, Mom, that's Mrs. Conlon. She's my nurse."

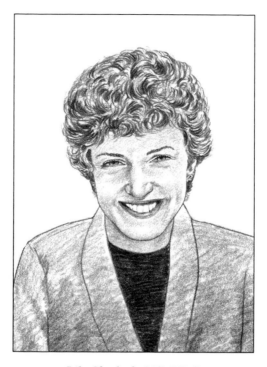

Lila Sherlock, MS, RN,C,
is a geriatrics nursing educator at the
Margaret Tietz Center for Nursing Care,
and a clinical associate at
Montefiore Medical Center,
Queens, New York.

The Nurse in Long-term Care

On the anniversary of her husband's death, a 90-year-old patient began telling me about her marriage. Her family had been opposed to the match, pressing her instead to marry someone who was better off. As a result she and her husband were forced to elope . . . on his motorcycle. The surprise and delight of exploring the histories of the very old opens up an entirely new perspective on life. It's one of the things that makes geriatrics nursing so interesting.

After graduating with a BSN in 1971, I worked in labor and delivery for nearly a year. After I married and moved to New Jersey, I worked as a public health nurse for two years. Later, I spent time in medical-surgical and occupational health nursing, and, after my daughter was born, I worked part time in Planned Parenthood clinics.

In 1980 I went to work in home care at Montefiore Hospital, and this provided my first extensive involvement with an elderly population. I worked as a home care coordinator, processing referrals from hospitals and community agencies and making initial home visits to evaluate patients for the "nursing home without walls," a long-term care program that enabled elderly people to remain at home with support services rather than entering a nursing home. Many of those referred to us were suffering from dementia and had been exhibiting behavior problems that presented a great challenge to management in the community. Through my contact with these people I developed an interest in dementia and its relationship to aging.

I had worked with nurse practitioners at Planned Parenthood and felt that was a role that I would find challenging and enjoyable. Consequently, I enrolled in a nurse practitioner program. Instead of concentrating only on geriatrics, I followed a broader track in adult care. I was invited to work at the Albert Einstein College of Medicine as a researcher on an arthritis study being funded through the National Institute on Aging (NIA). Two other investigations, one on falls and one on dementia, were being conducted at the time, and I also worked on the dementia study. In 1985, when I finished the nurse practitioner program, an intriguing opportunity was offered to me as a nurse practitioner in geriatrics. I also would work as a nurse educator in a nursing home that is affiliated with the hospital.

My duties at the nursing home were broadly defined to include education and research, and it was left to me to develop the specifics, working in collaboration with the staff at the facility and at Montefiore. One area of responsibility is in-service education. In addition to assisting with mandatory training on fire safety and accident prevention, I have conducted programs for staff on topics ranging from the normal aging process to strategies for dealing with stress. I obtained grant funding for Coping With Caring, a multidisciplinary program on understanding and managing demented residents. I also worked in collaboration with the assistant director of nursing to provide training designed to help nursing assistants obtain certification.

Most recently I've been involved in restraint-reduction rounds. This is an area of concern, because in U.S. institutions, it has been common practice to use physical restraints to prevent falls. Restraints are almost never used in European countries. The rounds focus on exploring alternative means of insuring resident safety.

I'm also currently engaged in research, including an NIA study on resistance to bathing in demented patients, and a New York State Department of Health project exploring whether the burden on family caregivers is relieved once the patient enters a nursing home. For some people, the pressure and stress are not alleviated, and the study focuses on some of the factors affecting the family adjustment.

Much of my time is now spent working with nursing assistants and RNs in the nursing home. Earlier, I had spent substantial amounts of time in nursing homes doing research, but I had not been involved in the day-to-day details of care in those facilities. As I began to interact with the caregiving staff I realized that practice in a nursing home is one of the least appreciated — and most challenging — of all nursing roles.

The head nurse in a long-term care facility has uncommon independence. Because a physician often is not immediately available for consultation, nursing judgement is a very significant element of patient care. This nurse must be a master planner, able to coordinate the efforts of all the personnel involved with a patient's care — from the attending physician to the charge nurse to aides and physical therapists. While a head nurse in a hospital works with a number of peers, the head nurse in a nursing home may be the only RN on the premises and one of the few full-time health care professionals there.

When new residents are admitted, the head nurse does an initial evaluation, including a physical assessment and detailed interviews that reveal the needs of each individual and the potential for independence in aspects of daily living. Using this information, the nurse, physician, and other members of the health care team develop a plan for care.

In addition to having physical problems, newly admitted nursing home patients often suffer from psychological or psychiatric disorders that affect their care. One of our residents, a woman in her 90s, was brought in by her son. She had been living alone but was becoming increasingly paranoid, a problem that was exacerbated by her hearing impairment and isolation. She thought her food was being poisoned. She was frail and could no longer care for herself properly, but because of her psychotic state, she refused to let anyone into the house to help her. Moreover, she refused to take medication that might have eased her paranoia. When her son and his wife brought her to the nursing home, the woman was enraged.

At first, she refused to eat, drink, or cooperate with her care in any way, so the nurses faced the monumental task of winning her trust. They gave her food in sealed containers as proof that it wasn't poisoned. Eventually, they convinced her that taking her medicine would make her feel less anxious. So she wouldn't feel she was being plotted against, they were meticulous about letting her know in advance what they were going to do. They worked with the nursing assistants to develop a consistent approach. By respecting her concerns, instead of attempting to force her compliance, the nursing staff were able to make enormous improvements in this patient's condition.

Dealing with family members is just as important as caring for the resident and, often, it is more problematic. The staff is faced with reconciling their practical here-and-now view of the resident with the family's emotional and historical perceptions of that person in his or her previous role of mother, father, husband, or wife. They must deal with the family members' feelings of grief and loss and help channel their unique knowledge of the resident's history into positive and useful information that makes it possible for the staff to give optimum individual care. Placing a relative in a nursing home produces predictable feelings of guilt. It also can engender financial worries and considerable friction among family members. The nursing staff works with family members, encouraging them to join support groups and helping them make their visits as positive as possible. Family members who have been caregivers struggle to the bitter end, and when they finally make the decision to place the person in a nursing home, they're frazzled and exhausted. By giving residents good physical care, the nurse is able to care both for the patient and the family, since then they're reassured that they made the right decision.

Nursing homes have suffered from a rather unsavory reputation, due in part to past scandals about facilities run exclusively for profit, neglecting the physical and psychological needs of patients. As a result, a tremendous amount of legislation governs the operation of nursing homes. Many of these regulations are admirable attempts to assess the need for care and to make certain it is available. The burden of documentation has increased significantly as a result of this regulation, however, and the nurse who has good verbal and written skills will find it easier to deal with the barrage of paperwork.

In the other part of my job, I function as a nurse practitioner, providing direct patient care through the hospital's geriatrics practice. My elderly patients live independently in the community and come to us for primary care. The practice includes attending physicians, fellows, nurse practitioners, and a social worker. In addition to providing patient care, each nurse practitioner has additional responsibilities. One nurse practitioner runs the home care program. Another manages education programs within the hospital, while I am involved with the nursing home.

At the hospital, for the most part, I deal with people who have stable chronic illnesses, including diabetes, cardiac problems, and dementia. I refer patients with more severe acute or complicated conditions to the physician. The problems I see here are similar to but usually less severe than those I see in the nursing home. The main difference is that clinic patients who live alone or are cared for by relatives often depend on my ability to coordinate aspects of their care with outside agencies and social workers. In that capacity, nurses who work in this field must be highly organized and resourceful.

In addition to the nursing home or a hospital's geriatrics unit, many geriatric care nurses work in a private practice with a physician. Others practice as visiting nurses or in day care programs for Alzheimer's patients. Still others work in life-care communities, in which elderly people live in their own apartments but have access to limited on-site health care facilities.

Geriatrics nursing is very rewarding. I enjoy being needed for emotional support as well as for physical care, and I enjoy the constant challenge of helping people maintain a balance between safety and independence. Working with the elderly requires an awareness of one's own attitudes about quality of life, right to die, and all the complex end-of-life decisions that modern medicine now presents.

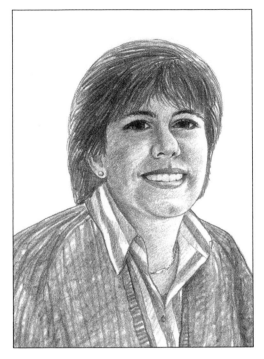

Greta Getlein, BSN, RN,
is a clinical supervisor at
Connecticut Hospice in
Branford, Connecticut.

The Hospice Nurse

Nurses and physicians are taught to save the patient, to work almost unquestioningly toward cures. If a patient dies, there is an implication that we failed — that we *lost* him. I used to hold that traditional viewpoint. But after three years of practice in an acute care setting, I began to have questions about death, dying, and the way we provide care.

In hospice, I found a completely different perspective, one that has more to do with life than death. Hospice gives dignity and comfort to terminally ill patients and their families. As a practice specialty, hospice is an environment in which nurses play a significant role in the provision and management of care. For me, hospice provided the answers I was looking for.

My introduction to hospice grew out of my experiences on a medical unit. I had been working on the unit for three years after graduation from nursing school. Most of our patients were suffering from kidney disease and renal failure. Our work was intense; patients were very sick and, in some cases, we could do little to make them better. We could help them die more slowly, but we could not prevent their death. Even so, a terminal prognosis wouldn't stop us from performing heroic resuscitative measures if the patient went into cardiac or respiratory failure.

For terminal patients who were in extreme pain, physicians prescribed morphine to help ease their suffering. In fact, during one month in 1989, I was the last person to administer morphine to three dying patients. All three died a few hours later — of the disease, not the drug. This was not uncommon, but it had never happened to me before. After each death I became quite upset and had long, emotional talks with my head nurse. She was helpful but wasn't able to give me the resolution I needed. I felt I had contributed to the death of my patients. I felt a sense of failure.

Soon after this experience, I discovered a grant-funded internship at Connecticut Hospice. I didn't know anything about hospice practice except that it focused on death and dying. But I reasoned that if anyone could help me think clearly about issues of death and dying, it would be these people.

During the week-long program I learned that hospice involves far more than simply waiting for patients to die. It concentrates more on life, and nurses who practice in this setting devote their efforts to making the life left to patients as comfortable and dignified as possible. A tremendous amount of attention is given to what the patients and their families want.

It was immediately apparent that hospice practice has more to do with patients than their diseases. Consequently, the care is very different from that at the hospital I worked in, where we were always scrambling to treat symptoms and conditions. On rounds, I saw a physician go from bed to bed, sitting down to talk with each patient. He didn't just ask a few questions and leave; he took time to really address each patient's concerns. At one bedside, the patient asked if the doctor thought the appearance of a new symptom meant the disease was progressing more rapidly. I knew from experience that such questions usually evoked broad, nonspecific answers. But the hospice physician was direct. He told the patient what the symptom meant and what would probably happen as a result. Then he explained the medical options. He was very specific and very honest. He did not assume that a certain plan of care would automatically be initiated. Instead, he asked what the patient wanted to do. No one at hospice lies to patients.

I was equally impressed by the independence with which hospice nurses practice. While the physicians provide diagnoses and write orders, actual management of patients is handled by nurses. Nurses confer with the physicians and coordinate a variety of services, including pharmacy, physical and occupational therapy, nutrition, and counseling. Nurses are permitted to challenge a physician's opinion and to discuss patient care as peers. While many hospitals have organizational structures that permit this type of exchange, they aren't taken as seriously as they are in hospice. If a hospice nurse disagrees with a physician's opinion, the physician never says, "Just do as I tell you." The more likely response is, "Why?" or "Okay, tell me what you think." There is a lot of give and take.

Nurses have a great deal of leeway in making decisions in this setting. They can't write orders for medications, but physicians write an order for a broad range of medications, giving the nurse discretion to choose drugs that are appropriate to the circumstances. For example, there usually are broad standing orders for managing fever, diarrhea, and various infections.

Throughout my internship, I kept saying to myself, "This is *real* nursing." After the week was over, I went back to my acute care practice, but I couldn't get the hospice out of my mind. I knew that was where I belonged. Within weeks I decided to leave my job and take a position at the hospice.

Most hospice services are home care programs administered independently or in cooperation with a hospital or a visiting nurse association. There are also hospice organizations, such as Connecticut Hospice, that combine home care with freestanding facilities. For a hospice to be certified by Medicare, it must provide around-the-clock on-call services, specialized medical equipment, and the ability to offer inpatient care. The federal government requires that four percent of all hours devoted to patient care be provided by volunteers. At Connecticut Hospice we have 200 paid staff members and over 400 volunteers.

Connecticut Hospice delivers care in three different settings: the patient's home, our own freestanding facility, and in a cottage that is owned by the hospice. Our home care is typical of that found in most hospice practices.

Home care is designed for patients who have progressive terminal illnesses, who have a prognosis of six or fewer months to live, and who are able to remain safely at home. Someone, usually a family member, must be available to care for the patient 24 hours a day. As a hospice nurse, I guide patients and their families through the home care process, managing the care and organizing services that may be needed. I act as the physician's eyes and ears in the home, assessing the patient's condition and the care being provided. I try to keep the patient fully informed so there won't be any surprises.

A first visit to the patient's home takes two or three hours. After that, I return two or more times a week, depending on what the patient requires. When I first enter a case, a great many services will be available to the patient. We want to help create and sustain a comfortable environment. If the patient wants to die at home, we do all we can to make that possible, including providing a full-time licensed nurse.

One of our main objectives in home care is balancing the components of care while trying to empower the families to become caregivers. As a result, about 80 percent of my practice involves teaching. Some of the focus is on physical care, such as how to give injections, change IVs, or bathe the patient in bed. We teach relatives to walk with the patient and how to transfer him to a chair or bed. In the beginning, there is plenty of help from aides and other services. But as family members learn what to do, we withdraw as many outside resources as we can. Even though family members are usually intimidated by the physical aspects of care, once they learn what to do, nearly everyone agrees it was easier than they expected.

The psychological aspects of death and dying command a great deal of emphasis. Many relatives are awkward and uncertain about how to act around a dying loved one. Often they feel they must always be doing something—fluffing up pillows, talking, holding the patient's hand ... something. But there are no rules, and I encourage them to relax, to sit or not sit, to talk or be silent, to laugh as well as cry. I have found that most patients accept their condition. It is the family members who really need the counseling and support.

Because the home care environment can be somewhat unpredictable, nurses carry a case load of about 10 patients and see an average of four per day. Some visits last 30 minutes, others take hours. For example, I recently spent two hours on what I thought would be a short visit. The patient was beginning to die, and his family had numerous questions for me about how the disease would progress and what they could expect during the next week or so. We spent a lot of time talking about how they were feeling and what they would need to do for themselves after the patient was gone.

While the basic philosophy of inpatient hospice care is similar to that of home care, there are some major differences. One is that most hospice inpatients have terminal illnesses with prognoses of two months or less, so they are generally much sicker than home care patients. Some are not that far along but have been admitted for a few days to treat a symptom or condition related to their disease. Others are there because there's no one at home to care for them, or because they have no home. The approach to care is the same as in home care, but more intensive. Inpatients receive 24-hour care from nurses and aides, and are seen by a physician every day.

Inpatient hospice is meant to reflect a home environment as much as possible. Floral patterns or bright prints usually replace white hospital sheets. In addition, patients are encouraged to bring in their own personal items — books and photographs, a favorite chair or lamp, and plants. At our inpatient facility, each room has a huge window that looks out onto a vista of green grass and trees. Because there are no set visiting hours, a patient's family and friends can come and go as if they were visiting at home.

As a practice setting, inpatient care can be emotionally challenging. In home care, the nurse spends only a couple of hours at a time with patients. Besides, these visits are separated by generous blocks of time spent traveling from one home to another. But in an inpatient hospice, the work is unrelieved for a full eight or 10 hours a day. Consequently, it is important for nurses and other staff members to have a support system. At Connecticut Hospice, we have regular times when providers get together to talk. We are permitted to eat lunch off premises. We also have what the nurses call our "screaming room," a small, sound-proof room with a soft chair and a large skylight. Nurses can go in there to talk, cry, think, or just relax. In recognition of the emotional toll our duties can exact, the hospice pays for an annual staff retreat.

We nurses are very good at taking care of each other, too. We talk things out and bolster each other emotionally. In fact, I've never before felt so supported by my peers. When I first began working here I noticed that other nurses were coming up to me and asking how I felt, or if I wanted to talk about what happened with a patient. I hated it — it was like being in therapy eight hours a day. But after a few months I realized how necessary it is. During my 15 months in inpatient care, I came to rely on this interaction.

Connecticut Hospice has a freestanding facility on the grounds that we call the *cottage*. This is a ranch-style home that houses five patients at a time. From a practice standpoint, the care we provide here is no different from home care; cottage patients either can't stay at their homes or have no homes. Currently, the facility is used for AIDS patients referred by local physicians and Yale-New Haven Hospital. Certified home health aides provide 24-hour care and a nurse makes regular visits.

In February 1993, I became a clinical supervisor for a satellite home care office we opened in another part of the state. We could coordinate these operations from the Branford facility, but we've found that being part of a local community makes a big difference in the way we are perceived by physicians, service providers, and patients and their families. In addition to coordinating and providing home care for local patients, I also make in-service presentations for area hospitals and nursing homes. I work with discharge planners, provide consults, and even do some marketing. These are new challenges, but I am enjoying myself. Almost everything I do involves teaching, which is the component of nursing that I like best. Many people still believe hospice is a form of euthanasia, that we just give people morphine until they die. This is frustrating to hear, but my new position gives me plenty of opportunities to tell people what we are really all about.

In hospice, death and dying are a constant reality, and it is difficult to work in this setting unless you have confronted your beliefs about these issues. For me, that was the hardest part of the practice. When I first began working here, I became so angry that I couldn't go to church for nearly four months. As a result of that period, I know how important it is for hospice nurses to balance their lives and be able to recharge themselves in their time away from practice. More than in any other setting I know, nurses in this practice who don't have some regular form of release and renewal face the near certainty of professional burnout.

As tough as it can be, there is something innately remarkable about hospice care. I love the feeling that comes with knowing I am helping people feel comfortable and worthwhile in the last months of their lives. I feel special when a family member thanks me, saying that I made this time less frightening than it might have been. To be frank, I can't imagine a career without hospice care.

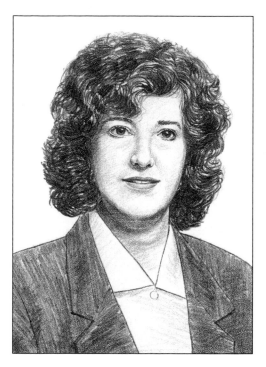

Trudy I. Reitz, MPH, RN, CNOR,
is director of operating room and
ambulatory surgery nursing at
St. Luke's/Roosevelt Hospital Center,
New York, New York.

The Operating Room Nurse

Many nurses are under the impression that operating room nursing is static, perhaps even boring. I think this impression is based on an assumption that we do the same things over and over again. Nothing could be further from the truth, because there are no constants in this specialty. Instead, this is a fast-paced, high-pressure practice that encompasses simple ambulatory surgeries and complicated bypass procedures. Patient presentations vary widely, and even patients being treated for the same condition may have completely different OR experiences. Nurses here have tremendous responsibility and have direct roles in a form of patient care that produces immediate results. This is not the formula for boredom.

The activities of OR nurses vary according to daily staffing needs. When they are circulating, they have responsibility for the preparation and safety of the patient and the management of the OR during surgery. In fact, the circulating nurse's responsibility begins even before the patient is brought into the preoperative area. The nurse reviews the chart of every patient in order to become familiar with the history and diagnosis. A plan of care is developed at this time. When the patient is brought to the suite, the circulating nurse introduces herself and carefully explains what can be expected, including a description of what patients will see and hear as they enter the OR, how they will be moved to the operating room table, and what procedures may take place before anesthesia is administered. We have found that knowing these details helps the patient attain a higher level of comfort and calm. Before entering the OR, the nurse goes through a checklist of safety-related information, including whether the patient wears dentures, has allergies, or has eaten within the past 12 hours.

After patients are brought into the room, the nurse helps the surgeon position them on the table and provides initial assistance to the anesthesiologist. Then the circulating nurse helps prepare the incision site and attaches safety straps and the return pad of the electrocautery unit.

The circulating nurse is the surgery patient's advocate. She constantly monitors events in the OR, making sure that sterility is not compromised. If the patient becomes unstable or goes into cardiac arrest, the nurse prepares emergency equipment and medications, and keeps the control desk informed of the progress of the procedure so preparations can be made for the next patient.

As manager of the case, the circulating nurse ensures that any necessary supplies are on hand. This professional handles tissue samples and specimens, making certain they are placed in the proper solutions, labeled, logged, and sent to the appropriate laboratory. The nurse also takes care of all documentation associated with each procedure: accounting for supplies, making entries in the OR log, cataloging samples and specimens, and maintaining sponge, needle, and instrument counts. After surgery, the circulating nurse helps prepare the patient for transfer to the postanesthesia care unit or recovery room, breaks down the room, restocks supplies, and begins preparing for the next case.

While the circulating nurse's job is to ensure the safety of the patient and the integrity of the OR, the assisting nurse provides direct aid to the surgeons throughout the procedure and manages all of the sterile equipment. Also known as the scrub nurse, the assisting nurse wears sterile attire throughout the procedure. Before the surgeons arrive, she sets up the table on which all of the surgical instruments are placed. Then she sees that any equipment to be used during the procedure is in place and functioning properly. When the surgeons arrive, she helps them gown and glove to ensure that sterile protocols are followed.

Once the procedure begins, the assisting nurse is the person who passes instruments to the physician. After they have been used, this person retrieves them, cleans and maintains them, and returns them to their proper field. In cases that involve an implant, the scrub nurse is responsible for preparing the implant according to specifications. This person also maintains medications used during the procedure, identifies specimens for the circulating nurse, and identifies which hospital lab will be receiving it. The scrub nurse also counts instruments, needles, and sponges before, during, and after the procedure.

In some hospitals, both the assisting nurse and circulating nurse make preoperative visits to the patient at the bedside to introduce themselves and tell the patient about the upcoming procedure. Then, a day or two after the procedure, the nurses return to see how the patient is doing. This visit provides an opportunity for the nurse to achieve some sort of closure with the patient. Such contact with patients puts a more human face on the practice.

The atmosphere in the operating room can be very stressful, but most OR nurses thrive on the pressure. It is a world of great precision, because surgical procedures are exact and extremely regimented right down to the way the instruments are arranged on the field. In fact, surgeons fill out preference cards that specify which instruments and sutures they prefer for each case. The physicians are intently focused, and this is reflected in the way they work. It is a changeable world, too, and the OR nurse must be able to react effectively in emergencies.

Once inside the patient, the surgeon may encounter a completely unexpected development and have to change the procedure radically. When this happens, the nurse must respond with the necessary medications, instruments, and equipment.

Errors, even seemingly small ones, are not taken lightly in the operating room, and this is no place for thin-skinned nurses. For instance, essential supplies may be hard to find if a sterilizer is broken or if central supply has let its inventory become depleted. Despite all the OR nurse does to get the supplies in time for the procedure, the surgeons may never acknowledge those efforts. This is just part of the job and should not be taken personally.

OR nursing is physically demanding—more so, in fact, than any bedside practice. The scrub nurse generally stands throughout the entire procedure, and some operations can last for many hours. In such cases, coverage may be available to relieve the nurse, but developments during surgery often make it impossible to take breaks. Standing for several consecutive hours during an intense surgical session makes a long day for anyone.

A major difference between OR nursing and other practices is that if the nurse disagrees with a physician in other settings, the issue can be discussed or argued or even brought to a third party for arbitration. There is no time for this in the OR, nor is there time for argument. The nurse must know her job and be assertive in carrying out her responsibilities, but she also must be able to manage her communications with other members of the surgical team.

Nurses are required to have at least a year of experience in medical-surgical nursing before they can be accepted in our OR training program. We have preceptors in every surgical specialty. After an initial phase of basic training, a nurse rotates through all services. In addition to providing specialized training, these preceptors act as mentors and advisors and make sure the nurse is acquiring skills at an acceptable level. Hospitals that do not have preceptor programs teach their OR nurses through extended on-the-job training programs. In either format, the nurses are not counted as OR staff until they are thoroughly proficient in procedures to which they are assigned.

Our initial training takes approximately three months, during which time nurses observe and participate in simple procedures in general, orthopedic, and gynecological surgery. They receive intensive instruction in aseptic technique and are taught to assist during surgery as scrub nurses. They also learn the management and patient care skills of the circulating nurse. At the end of this basic training, successful candidates enter a five-to-six-month period during which they rotate through more complex surgeries until they have experience in nearly every specialty. By now, they will have developed a moderate level of proficiency.

OR nursing is not for everyone. Our standards of performance are strict, and even though preceptors try to help candidates improve weak skills, some people simply are unable to achieve proficiency within what we consider an acceptable period of time. Some nurses recognize this and withdraw from the training; others we ask to leave. When that happens it's very difficult for everyone involved, but high standards have to be maintained in this practice.

For nurses who are interested in an OR practice, I recommend contacting a hospital's nursing department and setting up a time to talk with experienced OR nurses. Because it is so important to witness firsthand what it is like to work in this atmosphere, many hospital nursing departments will make arrangements for nurses to spend time in the OR. I believe that two or three days on the unit will give an interested nurse a feeling for this specialty.

For all its demands, OR nursing can be very satisfying. I enjoy anticipating the surgeon's needs and having the equipment and instruments ready when they're needed. I find a great deal of satisfaction in executing my responsibilities with the precision and the professionalism this setting requires. In addition, I enjoy the personal rewards that come from helping resolve a patient's problem. There is a remarkable clarity to that. Moreover, the operating room is a very intense environment that produces a strong feeling of camaraderie and collegiality among the team members.

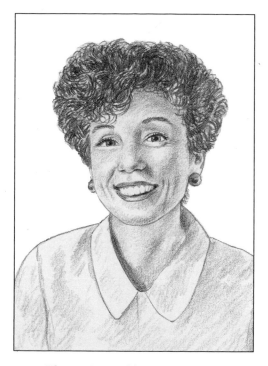

Theresa M. Doddato, MA, CRNA,
is director of the nurse anesthesia program
and associate dean of student affairs at
Columbia University School of Nursing,
New York, New York.

The Nurse Anesthetist

We have a saying in anesthesia. If everything goes as planned, the patient must have read the book. As a nurse anesthetist, I know how nice it is when that happens. The challenge of my job lies in integrating all the factors of a patient's physical and psychological state to select an appropriate anesthesia plan—then to know how to modify it during the actual procedure.

While I'm now on the faculty of Columbia University's School of Nursing as director of the nurse anesthesia program and associate dean of student affairs, I spent most of my career as a nurse anesthetist. I completed a diploma program in 1963, worked for a year as a medical-surgical staff nurse, and then spent another year as a clinical instructor. At the time, teaching wasn't right for me; I still wanted to do clinical work.

The mid-1960s saw the advent of the intensive care unit, a high-tech, dynamic environment that I found irresistibly appealing. I was able to find a job in the ICU unit, and I knew that I had found my niche. The equipment we used was state of the art, and every day I was getting training in physiology and pathophysiology. During my four years there, I became involved with the anesthesia department, initially because I went there for in-service education. I had never considered becoming a nurse anesthetist because, as did many other young nurses, I thought it was a scary job with an intimidating amount of responsibility. I believed it was best left to physicians. However, after four or five years, I matured and developed more confidence. When I realized that the time had come to get more education, I decided to become a nurse anesthetist, and I attended anesthesia school while completing my baccalaureate studies in biology.

Often, the nurse anesthetist's job begins the night before an operation, when the patient is given an introduction to what can be expected during the anesthetic procedure, as well as afterwards. Then the nurse reviews the patient's medical records and does a preoperative assessment of his or her condition, asking about previous experience with anesthesia as well as any medical or physical problems. At this time, the nurse discusses choices of anesthetic agents, listens to the patient's fears, and looks for conditions that could interfere with the anesthetic. For instance, the presence of cardiopulmonary disease or the use of certain medications will affect the choice of agents. In addition, the nurse anesthetist must understand details of the surgical procedure and be able to anticipate the likely effects of anesthesia during surgery.

191

Generally, the work day begins soon after 6 AM. Soon after that, the process of gathering the necessary equipment begins. For a major procedure, this might include sophisticated monitoring equipment as well as warming blankets, blood warmers, and other equipment needed to maintain homeostasis.

Before beginning to administer anesthesia, the nurse makes a last-minute check of the patient's blood pressure, pulse, and respiration, and then makes certain the respiratory support equipment is working properly. The nurse anesthetist must be compulsive. For example, I don't miss or forget things, because I do the same thing over and over again and never deviate from the pattern. In the OR, I go through a mental checklist, and I go through it very methodically: Is the patient breathing? Are the blood pressure and heart rate stable? It is a legal requirement that vital signs must be recorded every five minutes, but the nurse anesthetist knows them constantly. This information is used to adjust the depth of anesthesia and to prevent overdose. It is so easy to be distracted by activity in the operating room that the nurse pays little if any attention to the surgical procedure itself.

The physician-anesthesiologist is a collaborator and consultant, not merely a supervisor. And because this physician may not stay in the operating room, the nurse must be capable of working alone — sometimes under considerable pressure — while anticipating problems and developing contingency plans on a case-by-case basis. Each case is highly individual and there is no room for complacency.

I recall a patient who was undergoing lung surgery. She was very apprehensive and, in fact, had told me she didn't expect to survive the operation. She was about 55 years old and had a stable cardiovascular system, so there was no apparent reason for her concern. Still, just as the surgeon was closing, she went into cardiac arrest.

As I began to discontinue anesthesia and prepared to put the patient on 100-percent oxygen and supportive medications to get her blood pressure up, the physician was able to resuscitate her. Subsequently, an investigation into why she had a heart attack was initiated. We couldn't find a reason: It just happened. The lesson I learned was that if a patient says something is going to happen, don't dismiss the possibility.

As technology has advanced in the operating room, the nurse anesthetist's job has evolved to keep pace. Whereas we once monitored a patient's oxygen level by observing physical signs — skin and fingernail color, blood pressure, pulse — now, a small clip attached to the patient's finger immediately and precisely measures oxygen and carbon dioxide levels in the blood. That little device has revolutionized anesthesia, because it's made the process infinitely safer. Almost as readily, we can measure brain, muscle, and nerve functions. Technology may not have changed what anesthetists do, but it certainly has helped us do the job more precisely.

Administering anesthesia is a high-pressure job; there's no question about that. But as a career, it is almost perfectly suited for nurses because we are trained to be cautious and thorough. Mistakes hapen when people stop being vigilant.

While many nurse anesthetists work in acute care settings, there are growing opportunities in ambulatory surgery centers and in doctors' and dentists' offices. Also, many nurse anesthetists form group practices and contract with hospitals to provide service on an as-needed basis. Usually, nurses in this field work either in general anesthesia or in obstetrical anesthesia. The latter is a specialty in its own right because two patients are involved. Whatever is given the mother will affect the baby — and probably not in the same way. The obstetrics nurse anesthetist is especially knowledgeable about medical issues in pregnancy and is expert in fetal resuscitation.

Nurse anesthetists can design their work schedules with great flexibility, working as much or as little as they like — full time, part time, or on a per diem basis. Those who want work find plenty of it. In 1991, I served on an advisory committee that was commissioned by the federal government to determine the country's future need for nurse anesthetists. We concluded that meeting the demand for these specialists over the next 20 years will require a 40-percent growth in our ranks. I suspect that as health care reform draws attention to the high quality, cost-effective care provided by advanced practice nurses, that estimate may prove to be conservative. In addition to clinical work, there are teaching and administrative opportunities in this field.

Nurse anesthetists must pass certification boards, which they become eligible to take after graduating from a nurse anesthesia school, most of which offer two or two-and-a-half-year programs. Currently, a BSN is required, but by 1998, all programs must lead to a master's degree. Between one and two years of critical care experience are required for acceptance by most schools.

Besides having a compulsive nature, nurses who want to succeed in this fast-paced specialty must be able to handle a great deal of stress. The really good nurses can juggle several activities at once, spot problems before they develop into crises, and switch quickly to alternate courses of action. Here, you can expect to be given responsibility for the patient, so one of you must have read the book.

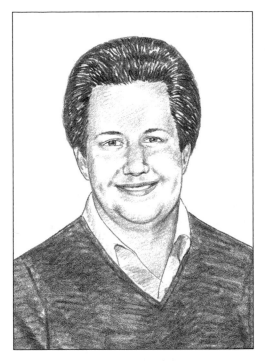

Harry E. Scher, MS, RN, CCRN,
is a staff nurse in the
medical intensive care unit at
Mount Sinai Medical Center in New York,
and an associate on the
clinical nursing faculty at the
Columbia University School of Nursing.

The Critical Care Nurse

Critical care nursing affords practitioners an array of professional practice opportunities that would be difficult to find in many other practice settings. Here, nurses enjoy high levels of autonomy and responsibility and regularly make important decisions regarding patient care. Our clinical skills are applied daily and often produce life-saving results. Because most critical care units use a collaborative practice model, nursing makes considerable contributions to the management of patient care. Moreover, nurses have extensive bedside interaction with patients and their families. Critical care nurses work with cutting-edge technology and treatment techniques.

My introduction to this field came about two and a half years after I began my nursing career. I was working in a Dallas hospital as a floater and was assigned to a different unit each day. As a result, I was exposed to an endless variety of practices and patient presentations. I experienced virtually every clinical nursing practice in the hospital — except critical care.

During the time I worked in this Dallas facility, it was suffering from a shortage of critical care nurses, as were many hospitals throughout the country. To solve its problem, the hospital began recruiting experienced nurses from within. When a supervisor asked if I would be interested in training for critical care, I was intrigued. I had heard other nurses talk about the challenges of this work, and I knew that with a patient-to-nurse ratio of two to one, it was possible to provide excellent care. I decided to accept the invitation and began my training. Within a week, I knew that I had made the best choice of my career.

What really hooked me was the high level of care patients required. They were extremely sick, often presenting with complex combinations of acute disease states and secondary conditions. All the skills I had acquired over the last two and half years weren't enough — I would have to become familiar with the latest medical technology and acquire a more extensive knowledge of pathophysiology, pharmacokinetics, and life-saving emergency protocols. But I liked the idea that I would be able to practice in an environment where my actions would have such an impact on patient outcomes. I also liked the variety of settings in which I could practice. At the time, I chose adult coronary care, but I could have opted for cardiac surgery, pediatrics, neonatology, or neurology.

The training program lasted six weeks and consisted of intense classroom instruction regarding the pathophysiology, typical complications, standard treatments, and expected outcomes of various disease processes. We also were given extensive training on the use and management of ventilators and other equipment. A large portion of the critical care course was devoted to the use of frequently administered medications. There was considerable emphasis on data analysis; critical care nurses read and interpret data generated by computers and monitors at the bedside and relate this to the patient's condition. Protocols, communicating with patients and family members, and interacting with other professionals on the unit also receive strong emphasis in training programs.

After completing the training, I started working on a critical care unit under the supervision of a preceptor. Intensive care unit nurses are regularly confronted with situations that require split-second assessments and immediate decisions. It is one thing to react perfectly in training conditions, but when it comes to real life, nothing seems to follow the textbook. A nurse's actions can mean life or death for the patient. For instance, if a patient has a seizure, the nurse must be able to recognize whether this is a result of the patient's condition, a drug reaction, or some other factor—and then react appropriately. Even when there's more time to act, the situation still may be volatile. For example, a patient with multiple intravenous drips may begin to demonstrate a slow but steady decline in vital signs. When this happens, the nurse may have to make a crucial adjustment, perhaps affecting blood pressure or cardiac output. Needless to say, it takes several months in actual practice to develop the experience and confidence required to feel comfortable in caring for the critically ill patient.

There's no end to the variety. Patients in the medical ICU present with everything from drug and alcohol overdoses to diabetic shock and severe respiratory failure. In any ICU the level of acute illness is high, but it is especially high in New York City hospitals, where there has been a shortage of ICU beds. By the time patients are admitted to the critical care setting, they are likely to be very unstable. Consequently, in addition to providing routine bedside care, I must monitor the patient minute to minute. Now, my assessment skills become crucial. Often, I can tell if something out of the ordinary is occurring, even if the monitoring equipment is showing no changes. It may sound like I'm claiming prescience, but the fact is that most experienced critical care nurses have developed their skills to such a degree that they can detect the most subtle changes in the patient's condition. In fact, most critical care nurses can tell if something is going wrong by simply looking at their patients. It's a valuable skill.

The care I provide is based on a collaborative practice model. This means that my assessments and the evaluations along with the observations provided by other members of the patient's care team all go into creating a plan for care. Because I spend the most time with the patient and am responsible for his day-to-day care, I coordinate all the specialties. Each day I meet with attending physicians, private physicians, allied health professionals, and other team members to discuss the progress of patients and the effects of our efforts. This approach gives the patient the benefit of many professional perspectives — all of which are aimed at the single goal of a positive outcome. In fact, recent studies show that such collaboration produces substantially better patient outcomes.

Because I have extensive interaction with other professionals, my communication skills must be sharp. It's not enough to report data and offer an interpretation of the patient's condition; I must be able to explain the meaning of the data from a nursing perspective so that physicians and other members of our team understand exactly what I mean. When we discuss strategies, I must be able to articulate my observations and beliefs convincingly. I also need to be able to listen critically when others explain their positions.

In dealing with patients and their families, the nurse must explain the condition, describe the treatments being employed, and make an appraisal of potential outcomes. In as much detail as possible, the nurse must make clear exactly what is going on with the patient and do so in a way that is neither condescending nor confusing. This can be an enormous challenge. The patient tends to be an easier audience. In fact, I have been repeatedly amazed by the dignity and calm with which people are able to accept their conditions, no matter how severe or life threatening. Relatives are another story, perhaps because of their anxiety over a loved one who is critically ill. Consequently, as liaison among the medical team, the patient, and the family, the nurse becomes educator, confidant, caregiver, and friend.

Unfortunately, dealing with death and dying is commonplace in the critical care setting, as many patients who enter an ICU will die. Usually, it is the nurse who must help families confront these issues. Often, this is an emotionally charged interaction. In some cases, as with AIDS and advanced cancers, we may have to discuss the appropriateness of "do not resuscitate" (DNR) orders that give the patient a chance to die with somewhat more dignity. These can be extremely difficult moments, especially if members of the family want to resist the requests of the patient.

Though we are empathetic and genuinely care about the patient, it is necessary to ensure that our own emotions and capabilities remain intact. Consequently, nurses who practice in critical care must learn to draw a line between professional involvement and emotional attachment to the patient. This detachment enables us to maintain a sense of balance and perspective in our lives. Nurses who cannot maintain this sense of balance will potentially burn out in a short period of time.

As tough as it is to lose a patient, it is even more frustrating to care for patients who are repeatedly noncompliant with their medical treatment. We often see young diabetics in the ICU who continually fail to follow their medical regimen. They are admitted with dangerously high blood glucose levels. We take care of these patients for several days, and then they spend another two or three days on a general medical floor before being discharged. Almost surely, they'll be back in a few months with the same problem. Not only are they hard to work with, but they are consuming resources that otherwise would be available to people with less opportunity for control over their illnesses.

Because of its many demands and high stress level, critical care nursing is not for everyone. People who are best suited to this type of practice thrive on pressure and seem to perform better as events become more intense. They are meticulously attentive to details and are confident in their clinical skills and assessment abilities. Effective communication skills are also essential for the ICU nurse.

At least one year of solid clinical experience is usually required before a hospital will consider a nurse for a critical care assignment. Aside from initial training and day-to-day experience on the unit, critical care nurses receive regular in-service education on new procedures, new equipment, and new modes of care. Certification in critical care nursing is offered through the American Association of Critical Care Nurses (AACN). The certification examination may be taken after one year of critical care practice. This exam is difficult and requires considerable preparation. While the CCRN certification is not required, it is a highly regarded credential.

Many critical care nurses spend their careers at the bedside. Most hospital intensive care units offer nurses three-day weeks with 12-hour shifts — a schedule that many nurses find appealing. Others become addicted to the excitement and challenge of providing this type of care. It is well that so many decide to stay because, currently, there is a significant nationwide shortage of critical care nurses.

For nurses who want to move into new areas, critical care experience is an excellent foundation for management, academics, consulting, and research. A critical care practice also can provide an excellent background for the nurse researcher. Currently, nursing research is being funded at a high level throughout the country. In fact, advances in critical care are increasingly the direct result of nursing research.

Make no mistake, this is one of the most demanding practice arenas in nursing. However, its rewards are unequalled in the profession. We have significant autonomy and tremendous influence as patient advocates. We provide comfort and dignity in the face of death, and we are able to make immediate, tangible differences in patients' lives. In my opinion, that's the best reward of all.

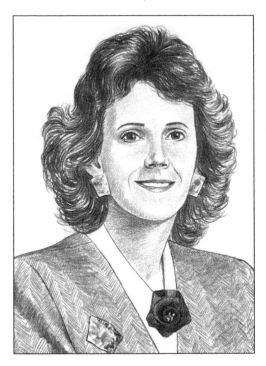

Susan Thomason, MN, RN, CS,
is a clinical nurse specialist in
spinal cord injury at James A. Heley
VA Hospital, Tampa, Florida.

Rehabilitation Nursing: The Inpatient Setting

As a clinical nurse specialist with a degree in advertising, my background isn't exactly par for the course. However, the advertising education has been helpful in communicating the many physical and psychosocial needs of persons with spinal cord injuries (SCI). Additionally, my advertising skills are put to work marketing our SCI programs in the hospital and the community.

I paid for my college education by working as a secretary in the orthopedics department at the medical school, a job that stimulated my interest in nursing. In fact, as soon as I received my baccalaureate degree in advertising in 1970, I entered nursing school. I completed my BSN studies in 1972.

At that point I took a job as a charge nurse in a general medical-surgical setting. Next I became a clinical instructor teaching medical-surgical nursing, but I found there was no place to go in academia with only a BSN. As a result, I decided to study for a master's degree in a clinical nurse specialist program. I graduated in 1975 as a medical-surgical clinical nurse specialist with a cardiovascular emphasis. Because I felt that lack of experience in critical care and ICU nursing was my Achilles heel, I took some critical care nursing courses and worked as a staff nurse. Even as a nurse with advanced training, I see the value in being a staff nurse, and at certain points in my career I've gone back to staff nursing to augment my skills and help further my career.

Because my husband was in the military, we traveled extensively, and I held several different jobs. I worked in home health in South Carolina, and taught medical-surgical and community health nursing at Rutgers University in New Jersey. I worked with the visiting nurse association and, when my husband was transferred to Germany, I worked as a school nurse and health educator. As a clinical nurse specialist, I had to market myself to facilitate the creation of some positions requiring my expertise.

When my husband retired, we returned to Florida, and in 1987 I took my current job working with persons who have spinal cord injuries. This is a class-I facility that is university affiliated, a circumstance that gives us a triple focus in clinical, educational, and research activities. The SCI department is a 70-bed service that delivers patient-centered, continuous care, beginning with inpatient treatment and continuing through outpatient care and clinic visits. I deal with outpatients only if there's a problem. For instance, I might consult with the staff about urinary drainage methods or the use of specialty beds.

The majority of my responsibilities are with inpatients, and I'm frequently called to consult on complex cases all over the hospital, whether they involve our spinal cord patients who have transferred to other floors, or medical patients with conditions that are related or common to spinal cord injuries.

For instance, I recently had to evaluate whether a diabetic patient in the ICU needed a specialty bed — a high-tech and high-ticket item. The patient was hypothermic and had numerous pressure ulcers. The bed regulates body temperature and through pulsating and floating motions relieves pressure on patients' skin, hastening healing. Working with an interdisciplinary team, I helped determine whether this patient's needs warranted the cost, and I recommended other care he might need. The nutritionist and I worked together to order dietary supplements that might help prevent pressure ulcers. Then, because the patient came in hypoglycemic, I worked with the social worker to determine whether he was getting adequate care at home, or whether his low blood sugar was related to substance abuse.

As chair of the SCI clinical practice committee, I have learned that other hospital departments need additional information to provide optimal care for persons with spinal cord injuries, so we developed a project to emphasize the physical and psychosocial aspects of caring for these persons. There are common myths about persons with SCI that I want to dispel. For instance, it is commonly thought that people with spinal cord injuries have no movement at all. In fact, the degree of movement depends on the severity of the injury. We may have quadriplegic patients who are less disabled than some paraplegics, because the injuries of the former are only partial.

Also, SCI patients may not lose sensation completely, and this should be a key factor when delivering care. While it is commonly perceived that SCI patients don't feel pain, many of them experience severe, debilitating, chronic pain. And, while many health care providers are inclined to treat pain with narcotics, SCI nurses are more aware of the potential for substance abuse and tend to work with other methods, such as spinal cord stimulation or medications to block the painful impulses. Another myth is that spinal cord patients must have permanent catheters. In fact, some can learn to void on their own, or they can be catheterized intermittently.

We're also teaching other hospital personnel about life-threatening complications that can arise, often within minutes, in an SCI patient. Autonomic dysreflexia, a complication that results from increased stimulation, as from a distended bladder or rectum, is such a condition. Without relief, this may provoke an exaggerated autonomic response and result in an extremely high blood pressure, retinal detachment, or heat failure. Nurses must know to look beyond obvious physical symptoms for potential problems. In consultation, we may suggest that patients with injuries above the sixth vertebra have bowel and bladder management strategies written into their care plans. However, while there are certain guidelines, there are no hard and fast rules about how to care for any patient's injury. Each one is individual.

Teaching is an important part of the job. Orientation of new staff involves a series of clinical and didactic classes that cover staff-patient relationships, rehabilitation theory, documentation, spinal cord injury medications, use of specialized equipment, psychosocial implications, urodynamics, care of new injuries, wound care, and many other topics.

A major aspect of SCI nursing involves general skin maintenance and care of pressure ulcers. As chair of the hospital's skin care committee, I teach extensively about these ulcers, which are often preventable. I emphasize the importance of turning every two hours, and periodically pushing up off the seat of the wheelchair to increase oxygen flow to the skin and relieve pressure. In addition, I work with other health care providers to pinpoint factors (incontinence, poor nutritional status, and substance abuse) that may exacerbate the condition. I also test new products that may help pressure ulcers and collaborate to develop protocols for prevention and treatment.

I strive to teach patients to achieve the highest possible level of self-care. I encourage them to take responsibility for themselves — to be directly involved in their own care, even to the extent of telling me what to do. Because turnover among their caregivers is so high, it's important that patients communicate their needs in order to ensure continuity of care.

When I teach patients, I follow up to make sure they are complying with instructions, and I serve as their advocate in securing any other services they need. It's important to remember that people with spinal cord injury can have all the problems of other patients. Therefore, we might have to treat concomitant diseases that may exacerbate the consequences of the spinal cord injury. For example, an SCI patient may not be able to use his coughing muscles, because injuries at the fourth cervical vertebra may damage the nerve that controls the diaphragm. This increases the risk of developing lung infections. In such cases, we teach other ways of coughing: a procedure similar to the Heimlich maneuver can be performed by a caregiver or by the patient.

Another facet of my professional life is serving on the editorial board of *SCI Nursing*, a refereed journal. As associate editor, I review manuscripts and try to facilitate publication by my colleagues.

Within the VA system, we're working to develop standards of care that apply to all SCI patients. Although there are exceptions to everything, such standards would cover details such as turning patients at prescribed intervals and performing bowel care according to a specific procedure. Now, we are working to computerize documentation of care, because this would make our records more complete and easier to access.

Besides standardization of care procedures, we're working on quality-improvement systems that would help us measure our success rate and concentrate on outcomes, because reimbursement procedures are likely to begin focusing more on ends than means. Even today, accountability is becoming a bigger and bigger issue in all areas of nursing. We can't look exclusively at process; we have to look at how things are affecting the patient. If the process doesn't work, we have to retool and find something that does.

The most frustrating aspect of my practice is dealing with patients who don't follow instructions. We can do everything for them in the hospital and teach them what to do when they go home, but the bottom line is that the effectiveness of their care depends on them. It's very frustrating to treat a patient, get his respiratory status cleared up, then see him again in two months because he's been smoking. To counter such compliance problems, we are increasing our educational efforts.

Because SCI nurses work with their patients on a long-term basis, we get to know them very well, and that's what is great about this field. We watch them progress through rehabilitation, and we see their transformation from complete dependence to self-sufficiency and productivity. We know we played a big part in this, and it's extremely rewarding to see the consequences of our interventions. All nursing is a potpourri of clinical and psychosocial skills, but nowhere is this mixture more important than in the rehabilitation of persons with spinal cord injuries.

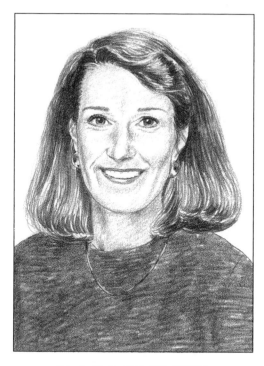

Linda Toth, MS, RN, CRRN,
is a clinical nurse specialist in the
spinal cord injury outpatient clinic
at the Department of Veterans Affairs
Medical Center,
Palo Alto, California.

Rehabilitation Nursing: The Outpatient Setting

During my early nursing career on a general rehabilitation medicine service I worked with patients who had various disabilities and neurological problems. Patients with spinal cord injury (SCI) are a distinct population; they fascinated me because their needs and care can be so complex and challenging. Spinal cord injury care entails respiratory, bladder, and bowel management, maintenance of skin integrity, dealing with the consequences of immobility, and determining psychosocial needs. These patients depend on top-quality nursing. For the past 10 years I have worked as a clinical nurse specialist (CNS) in an SCI outpatient clinic, and I still believe that caring for patients with spinal cord injury is the epitome of rehabilitation nursing.

When I received my BSN in 1971, I was positive I wanted to focus on intensive care or psychiatric nursing, but first I needed some general medical experience. My initial experience was as a staff nurse and later, as head nurse on a rehabilitation medicine unit.

In 1981, I returned to graduate school, and in 1983 I completed work on my master's degree. As a clinical nurse specialist in rehabilitation, I applied for my current position at the Veterans Affairs Medical Center in Palo Alto, California, as coordinator of the spinal cord injury service outpatient clinic.

The position I hold as a CNS had previously been filled by a nurse practitioner (NP). With my clinical and educational preparation and because NPs and CNSs share many common advanced practice skills, I felt prepared to assume the responsibilities of a CNS in an SCI outpatient setting. I brought with me experience in rehabilitation nursing with an SCI perspective, as well as physical and psychosocial assessment skills and management experience.

The SCI clinic is staffed by me, another CNS, and a physician who is the assistant chief of the SCI service. We are clinically and administratively responsible for approximately 1,000 patients. Initial contact occurs when patients are admitted to the hospital. Then, we follow them through their acute rehabilitation and provide follow-up as they reenter the community. In this way, we serve as primary care and managed care providers.

As a primary care and managed care provider, the CNS works with the multidisciplinary team to manage and guide the individual with SCI through a continuum of health care services and community resources. We must ensure that care is coordinated, accessible, and comprehensive and that continuity and follow-up are provided. The CNS provides support and advocacy for the person with a spinal cord injury.

Because we know our patients and their families so well, and because they feel comfortable with us, the clinic is managed rather informally on a professional and comprehensive yet personal basis. Our staff is extremely experienced, and we are thoroughly familiar with all patients — from their medical histories to details of their family and community involvement.

Outpatients are generally scheduled at six-to-12-month intervals for SCI and primary care checkups. The SCI center covers a large geographic area, and patients may live several hours away, so we try to preplan in order to accomplish as much as possible during each visit. This may include a general physical examination, urological evaluation, EKG, chest x-ray, and laboratory work. SCI patients are at high risk for developing renal and urological complications, and we constantly monitor for these problems. Other interventions during this visit may include an equipment and wheelchair evaluation by an occupational therapist, a physical therapy evaluation, a dietary consultation, or a meeting with the psychosocial staff.

Much of our work is focused on prevention. Due to impaired sensation and mobility, persons with SCI are at increased risk for developing pressure sores. We teach techniques that assist in maintaining skin integrity (eg, pressure relief), positioning, and using protective devices.

Respiratory complications are also common in individuals with spinal cord injury. In severe cases, ventilatory support may be required. Some patients are unable to breathe deeply or cough naturally, and this increases their susceptibility to pulmonary infections, including pneumonia. To prevent complications, we teach specific breathing and coughing techniques.

In addition to routine wellness checkups, patients often present to the SCI clinic with specific problems. An example might be onset of sweating, chills, and cloudy, foul urine. In this circumstance we take vital signs and a careful history, and we perform a thorough physical examination, urinalysis, urine culture, and other pertinent laboratory work. With physicians' consultation, a diagnosis of urinary tract infection might be made and an appropriate antibiotic course prescribed. We would then need to determine why the infection occurred. I would not be surprised to learn that the patient had recently taken a long airplane trip during which time fluid consumption was decreased. This could explain the infection, and we would need to discuss with the patient the importance of complying with recommendations for bladder management. If infections were recurrent, a further diagnostic work-up would be indicated.

In this setting, it is extremely important to remember that we are treating the whole person, not just the spinal cord injury. If a patient presents with a cardiac or endocrine problem, we are responsible for appropriate treatment and/or referral. People with SCI live full life spans and therefore face the same problems and chonic illnesses of aging as the general population.

We also coordinate specialty clinics that address specific problems experienced by persons with SCI. For example, the SCI upper-extremity clinic is staffed by plastic and orthopedic surgeons who specialize in correcting hand and shoulder dysfunctions and tendon-transfer surgery to enhance hand function for quadriplegic patients. Our occupational and physical therapists work closely with us in this clinic. Also, because patients with SCI are susceptible to problems associated with hypercoagulation, we coordinate a weekly SCI coagulation clinic.

Fifty or so patients are seen each week, and others may have telephone consultations. In this way, we are able to deal with various patient questions and problems and to consult with care providers in the community and colleagues in other facilities.

Helping patients adjust to their changed social and home circumstances is a challenging part of this job. If a patient requires a special diet, it is easy enough to teach why this is necessary. However, because a spouse may do the shopping and cooking, she or he also must be educated. Or, suppose the patient is a young man who has become quadriplegic after being injured in a construction accident. The life of his wife and young children will be affected, too. Previously, the wife may have stayed at home to care for the children, but now she may need to assume financial responsibility and return to work. In a situation such as this, the entire multidisciplinary team would intervene to assist and support the family in adaptation and role adjustments. As part of this process, the family's psychosocial needs and educational and vocational resources would be assessed and addressed. Our aim is to do everything possible to assist the patient in developing the self-confidence and skills needed to function successfully in the family and community.

Education, encouragement, and reinforcement are the underpinnings of work in SCI rehabilitation. This is an extremely stressful period for the patient and family; they are frightened and are being bombarded with information they may not fully comprehend. Our job is to teach them what they need to know and reinforce it until it becomes second nature. We try to provide support to patients and their families so they don't give up.

In my CNS role, I was active in the development of our center's peer resource network, a program in which individuals who have been injured for some time serve as resources for patients with recent injuries. They share their own experiences — describing how they coped and adjusted — with patients, spouses, and other family members. As nurses, we can discuss what we know about spinal cord injury, but we know that people learn best from those who have been through similar experiences.

Beyond my clinical responsibilities, I am active in the American Association of Spinal Cord Injury Nurses and other professional organizations. I serve on the editorial board of *SCI Nursing* and enjoy publishing and participating in nursing research. I also am involved in promoting wheelchair sports and coordinating related activities, including the National Veterans Wheelchair Sports Program and the National Triathlon for the Physically Challenged. These activities, in addition to my daily practice, enhance my professional experience and satisfaction.

Perseverance and continuing vigilance are of utmost importance for individuals with spinal cord injury. These are the survivors of disability. As nurses, we must share what we know, learn from our patients, and provide mutual support.

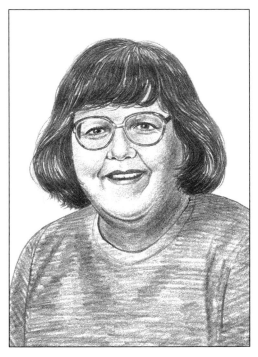

Mary Martin, BSN, RN,
is head nurse in the special treatment unit
for spinal cord injury at the
Department of Veterans Affairs
Medical Center, Long Beach, California.

Rehabilitation Nursing: Managing Chemical Dependence

In my professional career I've developed an appreciation for the fact that no one wants to be chemically addicted. Addicts don't use drugs to feel wonderful; they use them just to feel okay. Chemically dependent people don't seek help until the pain of using becomes greater than the pain of not using. As the head nurse in a chemical dependency unit for spinal cord injury (SCI) patients, I do double duty. I help people overcome their drug dependencies — a job often made more difficult because of their injuries — and I work on rehabilitation issues that were ignored when the person was chemically dependent.

I graduated from a diploma nursing program in 1959, then received a BSN from Marquette University in 1963. For a year after that, I worked for a county hospital, then moved to California in 1964. In 1966, and after working in a private hospital for a couple of years in areas from orthopedics to pediatrics, I came to the Long Beach Veterans Affairs Medical Center (VAMC). Working at the Long Beach VA was my first experience working with SCI patients.

I've always been attracted to the challenge of working with the more difficult patients — those who are angrier or making less progress in their rehabilitation. I don't look at these patients as bad or weak people. I see them as people who have problems in their lives that prevent them from achieving maximum mental and physical potential. As a nurse, I believe in sitting down with them — individually and in groups — and talking through the issues. I try to cultivate a spirit of cooperation. This is a fairly straightforward philosophy, but it can have incredible results. For example, one of our patients isolated himself from both the staff and other patients. Yet after I worked with him for a while, his attitude changed sufficiently that I was able to elicit his participation in a small way: I got him to make his bed. It was a little thing, but it signified his willingness to respond to others and begin taking responsibility for himself.

In rehabilitation, it's particularly important to make patients feel involved with their own care and rehabilitation. Over the long term, our goal is to help patients acquire new capabilities, despite their limitations. As a result, we teach computer skills, and we have an incentive program in which patients are paid for work they do in the hospital. I enjoy the challenge of meeting the needs of tougher patients, and, more to the point, the challenge of teaching those patients to meet their own needs.

When spinal cord injuries are complicated by chemical dependence, the result is just that kind of challenge. However, the plan of care for a chemically dependent person with such an injury is not different from the plan of care for a chemically dependent person who is not injured. The difference lies in the care environment. Here, spinal cord injury is a common denominator—all the patients share this disability, and the nurses are well acquainted with the consequences. This serves as a bond for the patients in group therapy, and it makes it difficult for them to manipulate others by soliciting pity.

Accountability is important for these patients, because it is common for society to excuse handicapped people and not hold them responsible for their actions. For example, an ordinary person who is arrested for drunk driving is more likely to get tossed in jail than a disabled person, who might inspire lenience from a judge. Unfortunately, this clemency compromises the rehabilitation process. As long as a person is relieved of responsibility for his actions, as long as his pain is assumed by others, then he will not reach the critical threshold where the pain of his using becomes greater than the pain of not using.

When patients finally come to us, it's because the chemicals have stopped working, and they're miserable even when they do use them. Their personal relationships and family support systems have fallen apart. They may be without money or in trouble with the law. They've stopped managing their lives and are ignoring their rehabilitation. They've stopped caring and they no longer are acting as their own advocates.

Chemical dependence usually stems from ineffective coping, so once we get patients physically free of chemicals, we still have to help them face the issues in their lives. They may act arrogant, but they sure don't feel that way. On a scale of self-confidence, a person who checks himself into a chemical dependency unit — spinal cord injury or not — ranks very low. Therefore, one of the biggest challenges for a nurse in this field is to foster feelings of self-worth and self-esteem among patients who have hit rock bottom.

If a patient begins performing his bowel care at three o'clock in the morning in order to obtain more privacy, it may be that he is having problems with his body image. Having noticed this, the nurse should help the person confront the issue. Many drug abusers had negative images of themselves even before they were injured, and the injury compounds the problem. The nurse steps in by helping the individual perform self-care with increased feelings of control and, thus, an improved self-image.

As patients begin to deal with psychosocial issues that were ignored or blocked by drugs, the nursing staff must know how to direct their behavior appropriately. For instance, if the nurse talks with a patient in the middle of the night about his fears and concerns, that frees him from talking about those problems during group therapy, which is a more productive time. Also, it's not uncommon for patients to ask to leave — to go to the bathroom, for instance — during group therapy as a way of avoiding painful situations. We don't allow that. The reason so many people with SCI do not do well in outpatient programs is that they're never confronted with their behavior and, consequently, never have to confront their own feelings.

Nurses should serve as socialization models for patients, talking and interacting with them in ways that teach appropriate forms of communication. Rehabilitation, in a sense, is learning to mirror the public. Rather than allow a patient to be ostracized and lonely, it's important for the nurse to tell him his behavior is unacceptable. For instance, if a patient makes a sexually inappropriate remark, the nurse should say, "That was a sexually inappropriate remark," not call the patient a dirty old man and walk off in a huff. Chemically dependent people almost always come from dysfunctional families in which they were subjected to humiliation. We should not add to that. Instead, we have to demonstrate and explain appropriate behavior that respects other people's feelings.

In another example of designing constructive communication systems, we have established community meetings for patients, thereby creating a kind of government that lets them determine aspects of their lives, such as where they will go on their weekly outing, and gives them a forum for registering complaints or compliments.

While nurses should help patients and facilitate their rehabilitation, they must always maintain a professional distance. It is important to draw a line between being an advocate for the patient, and contributing to his dependency. Nurses are naturally very caring people, but they must be careful not to do for the patient instead of encouraging independence. Nurses in this practice must learn not to equate being needed with being wanted and to understand that personal relationships with patients are inappropriate. Observing the ethical boundaries of the profession is important in every area of nursing, but it is especially important in long-term rehabilitation. It is vitally important with substance abusers who are looking for someone to manage their lives.

The desire to help someone who is suffering is strong, and it's easy to step beyond the limits that will help the person reach for self-sufficiency. That's why it helps to work as part of a multidisciplinary team that includes nurses, social workers, psychiatrists, and therapists. If any member of the team is particularly sympathetic to a patient and is inclined to extend special concessions, the other members force that person to look at the facts.

We meet every morning to talk about our patients — 10 inpatients and 10 outpatients — and about issues affecting their care. Also, we meet with each patient every two weeks to set goals. In the room where we hold those meetings there is a communication board on which patients write questions or express their concerns. We may see a note indicating that a patient came back early from his Alcoholics Anonymous meeting and looked anxious, or that another patient didn't sleep well. Even if a patient skips dinner, we want to know about it, so we can be on the lookout for possible problems. This is the place to ask questions, vent concerns, and disseminate information to the rest of the staff.

A plan for nursing care is formulated by a patient's primary nurse, based on a nursing assessment that considers educational, environmental, discharge planning, and other self-care factors. The plan is designed to address a hierarchy of problems, such as powerlessness and depression. Manipulative behavior is also common in drug-dependent SCI patients, so nurses limit the potential for this behavior. The plan should help patients consolidate and direct their own care. Consolidation of care helps because it conditions patients not to ask for something every five minutes. Even more important is direction of care, because this empowers patients to take control of their bodies and their lives.

Never underestimate structure as a form of therapy: That's an important saying in this unit. We deal with patients whose lives have become chaotic, so we run a very structured ward. The nurses set parameters and guide patients through those parameters 24 hours a day. We provide SCI care within a drug therapy plan, and patients and nurses alike always know what will happen and when. We create a therapeutic milieu for patients, but because this is participatory recovery, the patients must be included in the work.

As head nurse, it's my job to create an environment that enables my staff to manage complex problems. I listen, guide, interact, am receptive, and share ideas. A large part of my work involves teaching, and my goal is to teach the staff every time I talk to them. I'm in charge of quality assurance and, drawing on my general rehab background, I may work with patients on other units who are presenting challenges. In addition, I've volunteered my time to work with an alcoholism advisory board that works to get drug and alcohol treatment for disenfranchised populations, such as adolescents or the elderly.

It's wonderful when I can help patients and make a change in their lives. However, I never forget that it's the patient's prerogative to go out and begin using chemicals again. I don't have to like that, but I can't prevent it. We have to remember that human beings have the right to make their own choices.

I hand-pick my staff, and for this job I look for nurses who are working hard to improve themselves as nurses and as human beings. I look for people who are willing to change and to learn as the job requires. People who work here have to be able to say no, but they have to say it in an encouraging way. I want nurses who can combine the traditional caregiving duties of rehabilitation — performing bowel care or taking care of pressure ulcers — with a psychiatric component. Most of all, I want someone who will treat patients with the respect they deserve as human beings. The plea I've heard over and over from SCI patients is that they just want to be treated like everyone else. I think that's fair.

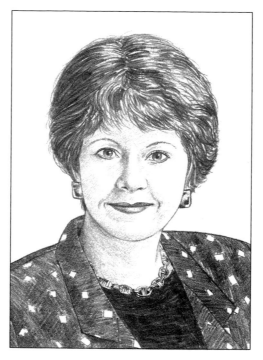

*Katharyn May, DNSc, RN, FAAN,
is professor and associate dean for research,
and director of the PhD in Nursing
Science Program, Vanderbilt University
School of Nursing,
Nashville, Tennessee.*

The Nurse in Academia

My term papers were coming back with A's on them, but red ink was dripping out of the margins. I was working on my master's in maternity nursing, and my adviser was trying to tell me something. I finally understood her plan when she returned my third revision of one paper and suggested I submit it for publication. I did, and when it was published in the *Journal of Obstetric, Gynecologic, and Neonatal Nursing* I realized I had a potential for intellectual work. That was a turning point in my life.

Before, as a starry-eyed girl out to save the world, I saw myself as an activist in nursing—academia was not part of my plan. I had graduated from Duke with a double major in nursing and psychology, and my sights were set on nurse midwifery. But when I went for my master's degree at the University of California, San Francisco (UCSF), my adviser started marking up my term papers and pointing out, not very subtly, that my clinical skills were average, but my academic ones were outstanding.

As I was finishing my master's work I became interested in the male partner's effects on pregnancy. I wanted to extend my master's program to explore that subject, but I couldn't enlist the support of my advisers. When I asked why, I was told bluntly that it was foolish for a master's student to struggle through a research project. Why not enroll in the doctoral program and do it right? So, at age 25, I did.

The doctoral program drew on all my background—from psychology to prenatal care, and I realized that I loved the world of ideas. I wanted to work with clinicians and thinkers alike, and I wanted—the 1960s girl in me at work—to push back the barriers of ignorance. I had jumped into the doctoral program to do research, but most of the opportunities for doctorate-level nurses were, and still are, as professors in schools of nursing. Fortunately, when I completed my doctorate of nursing science in 1978, a tenure-track position opened up at UCSF. I was thrilled to get it, because I knew UCSF was oriented to research and that my first love would be high on the list of my responsibilities. Of course, I also had to be a good teacher.

Teaching is extremely rewarding and extremely difficult. I was better in the classroom than in a clinical setting because my gift lay in being able to help people refine their ideas. With tenure in mind, I planned my next five years carefully. While teaching obstetric nursing to undergraduate students, I also conducted small studies on expectant fatherhood in order to get my research career off the ground.

As is true in any career, becoming an established academic in the field of nursing has certain benchmarks. First, it's necessary to become established as a working scientist in an area where the requirements for success boil down to one's ability to publish and attract research funds. This creates a quandary: It is necessary to perform research in order to write, and it is necessary to have published work in order to attract research money. I was fortunate to find a mentor who was already conducting funded research.

As was carefully spelled out to me at UCSF, I had six years to make tenure. In that time, I needed at least two data-based publications a year, preferably more. I also had to get seed-money grants for small research projects. Then, within three or four years, I had to start applying for NIH funds, the primary source of federal funding. Research and publications lead naturally to the third criterion for a successful academic — a national reputation.

In time, I published *Comprehensive Maternity Nursing*, a textbook that became a leading resource in this field for BSN students. Some in academia avoid writing textbooks. They reason that the effort counts no more than does an article in their publication credits column, despite the additional investment of time. Moreover, it's not necessarily considered a pinnacle of intellectual achievement. However, I believe that writing is an extension of my teaching role, and I wanted to write a textbook that emphasized what I thought was important, which is a holistic approach to patient care. During my first three years at UCSF, I taught a two-hour undergraduate lecture course that entailed two days in a clinical setting with students each week and two days in preparation for class or taking care of administrative chores. The fifth day I spent on writing or research. After my third year I began teaching in the graduate program, and my classroom load increased to about five or six hours a week. By then, I was spending two and a half to three days with students.

The 60-hour week is alive and well in academia. When I first considered an academic career, I envisioned long, contemplative afternoons in the library. Instead, I've become a speed reader par excellence, because academics can't allow themselves to get sloppy in their professional reading. If they do, they soon find that their research doesn't get funded and their students know more than they do.

I developed my academic specialty by studying a topic that fascinated me, and I was lucky to find myself in an environment that supported my passion. Then, as I did more research, my interest broadened until it encompassed something I could teach. I am primarily a scientist and am driven by a desire to know more about childbearing families. Whenever possible, I try to merge my research and teaching. For instance, I now teach "Inquiry in Nursing," a course that explores ways advanced practice nurses can use research. Other nurse academicians are not as driven by science as I am, but they may be crafting their careers differently. Their research may be more closely related to their clinical practices, while I ask more abstract questions with broader implications.

Asking relevant questions when I'm not in a clinical setting requires that I maintain relationships with expert clinicians. As a result, I've assembled an inner circle that meets regularly for lunch to keep me up to date on clinical issues. In the process I've cultivated very good listening skills and have become skilled at drawing information out of my colleagues.

I spent nine years at UCSF. When my mentor retired in 1987, I came to Vanderbilt University to chair the department of family and community nursing. I signed on for five years — no longer, because I think it's important that a faculty not become too dependent on a department chairman. When I took the job, I was interested in recruiting good people to improve the school of nursing. I also wanted to attract my own research money and build a doctoral program, of which I became the director in 1992.

As department chairman, I had direct responsibility for my faculty members. I made teaching assignments, consulted on course design, prepared the department budget, and worked with the faculty to establish new directions for the school. For instance, while Vanderbilt had a nurse practitioner program, we didn't have clinical settings that we controlled. Now we do. While I wasn't directly involved in establishing them, I was instrumental in the idea process.

As director of the doctoral program, I teach graduate students and research courses exclusively. I'll tell you this: The best part of my job is watching students' eyes light up with excitement. Seeing that happen in even one student in 30 motivates me for several weeks.

About the time I came to Vanderbilt, I became a fellow in the American Academy of Nursing (AAN), which functions as a nursing think tank. Members are elected based on their contributions to nursing, as well as their potential for continuing contribution. As a member of the health policy committee, I helped write position papers about nursing care for women and children. The AAN is crucial for academic nurses. This network of accomplished nurses helps keep the academic challenge fresh and exciting.

Currently, academic nursing is in flux. It is shifting rather dramatically toward a requirement that educators hold doctorates. Unfortunately, many nurses today pursue doctorates not because they want to, but because they feel they must. And nothing ruins a master's-prepared star clinician faster than pursuing a doctorate for the wrong reasons. It should not be done for the money, because a master's-prepared nurse specialist can easily top an academic's salary of $50,000 to $75,000 a year.

The field of nursing needs both master clinicians and scientists. Indeed, in intermingling the skills of both lies the future of nursing education. But we're not there yet. Although I'm in favor of nurses pursuing doctoral degrees, nursing schools now need to attract master's-prepared expert clinicians to teach. Our profession has come to realize and accept that it can't have clinical teachers who are not actively working in clinical settings. Academic nursing, therefore, is seeking ways to help people maintain their clinical talents while enhancing their research skills. At Vanderbilt, we've experimented with ways to let clinicians balance their teaching and practice responsibilities. Split positions between academic and clinical settings (sometimes involving a split salary) are one solution. In addition, we have a clinical faculty track that allows nurses to rise through the professorial ranks on the basis of clinical and teaching experience.

Unfortunately, at many schools of nursing, the faculty not only are not engaged in science, but they're not even engaged in practice. This may reflect a lack of desire, and it may be because it's difficult to find a school that will support a combination schedule. But it's a fairly typical situation, and it is of some concern in academic nursing. Nevertheless, the situation is changing. Fifteen years ago, when I was a graduate student, I didn't know any faculty who were in practice.

I think the path I followed to academia is still, with modifications, a good one. Because I spent little time in practice, I have to overcompensate in that department. My clinical experience is limited to work as a patient care technician in labor and delivery for three years while I was in nursing school and a brief position in postpartum and nursery care as a graduate student. For students interested in an academic career, I recommend working as a staff nurse for two or three years after getting a BSN. Next, choose a specialty and find a good master's program that offers access to a doctorate track. Either move directly from the master's into the doctoral program, or take two or three years to work after earning the master's degree. But don't wait too long before going back for a doctorate.

I'd like to see more nurses get their doctorates in their early 30s. In fact, the average age of entry into a doctorate program in nursing is dropping fast. It used to be that nurses would establish themselves in academia, go back for a doctorate in mid-life, and have 15 years in a postdoctoral career. Now they're entering in their 20s and expecting to enjoy 35 years of postdoctoral work. That trend will undoubtedly affect the character of nursing research. Instead of small studies, we'll begin to see well-developed research programs producing significant bodies of work.

Nurses who choose an environment where the teaching load is heavy should be aware of changes we are seeing among students. For one thing, we are beginning to get students who don't read well and who have television-inspired attention spans. For another, there are increasing numbers of minority and male students, and faculty will have to adjust as cultural diversity hits nursing.

Changes in the U.S. health care environment are certain to redefine nursing. As a result, nursing academics must be prepared to adapt our curricula to meet the challenge of the future. We may have to prepare our graduates to work in fields that don't even exist yet.

While anticipating the future, nurses in academia also must work to bring the nursing profession completely into the present. Most notably, we must stop allowing nursing to be an undervalued profession. One of the most frustrating aspects of my position is dealing with the lack of recognition accorded nursing. I plan to change that however I can. In fact, I'm just waiting for the day a nurse wins the Nobel Prize.

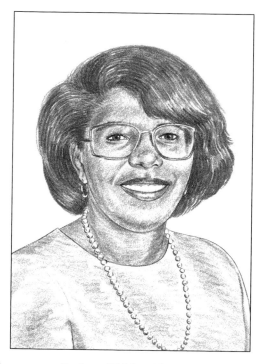

Barbara Holder, PhD, RN,
is an associate professor at the
New York University School of Nursing,
and an adjunct professor at
George Washington University,
Washington, D.C.

The Nurse in Research

Many nurses are intimidated by the prospect of a career in research. This is unfortunate because research is nothing more than asking questions and looking for answers. It is doubly regrettable because nurses are so well suited by their education to conduct research. I was more than a little anxious when I began my own clinical research activities over 10 years ago. But any lack of confidence I had quickly gave way to the intrigue and pleasure of inquiry and resolution.

My work has focused on health problems among African Americans: specifically the elderly with diabetes and those with renal disorders requiring dialysis. I also study mental health problems that occur among patients and their families in both groups.

I became interested in these patients during the 1960s when I was practicing at an ambulatory care clinic in the Bedford Stuyvesant section of Brooklyn. I had been attracted to community health nursing because my mother was an active proponent of improving health in our community. Together with her contagious enthusiasm, my own concerns as a mother in the neighborhood were more than enough to bring me into that practice. However, it was at this point that I began asking the questions that led me into research.

The clinic provided medical as well as mental health care. And because I had undergraduate training in mental health I worked in both areas. Over the course of a few months, I began to notice that many patients who came in for treatment of chronic medical problems were also patients of the mental health service. I wondered whether there might be correlations between the two—if certain systemic disease states predisposed patients to mental health problems, or vice versa.

I was equally curious about elderly African-American patients with diabetes. Of all populations, African Americans have one of the highest rates of diabetes. The problem was particularly severe among the elderly in our clinic. These patients experienced higher rates of blindness and had to have more amputations than diabetes patients in other populations. Exposure to this was quite upsetting, but it made me want to know more about the disease and why its effects are so severe among these people. I searched the literature, but the information to be found on African-American patients told me little that I didn't already know.

I realized that if I wanted to do more for these patients, I would need more training. As a result, I decided to get a master's degree, which I knew would provide the specialized knowledge, skills, and credentials I needed for an advanced practice. What I did not anticipate was that it would also give me a chance to begin answering the questions I had been asking.

During my studies, I became aware that nurses were involved in research at a number of levels — as data gatherers, coinvestigators, and principal investigators. I don't think I related this to my own career until I took a course in research and research methods. Then I saw how fascinating the world of research can be. I mentioned my excitement to my mentor, Dr. Hattie Besset, and she encouraged me to pursue the interest. She told me that if I were a researcher, I wouldn't have to wait for others to address the questions that had been bothering me. She even helped me find funding for my PhD studies.

It is impossible to overstate the importance of having mentors. I use the plural because it usually is necessary to have more than one. The guidance of one individual may be significant, but is apt to be limited to one area or to a single aspect of a person's interest. Others may have a life-long impact. I have learned more from some mentors than others, but each relationship has its own value.

One of the questions I get from undergraduate and graduate nursing students is: How do I find a mentor? In truth, most find you. An instructor or expert may begin offering increased attention or assistance to a student who shows unusual enthusiasm or insight. Don't be afraid to acknowledge such encouragement, because it could signal the beginning of a rewarding professional relationship. But don't sit around waiting for this kind of interest to develop, either. The most direct way to acquire a mentor is to identify a person whose experience coincides with your own aspirations, and ask for a mentoring relationship. Before asking, though, make sure this is an expert from whom you can truly learn. Become familiar with this person's body of work. Remember, effective mentors are intensely devoted to their careers. It is a good bet that if you are knowledgeable about a prospective mentor's work and explain your own goals, a relationship is possible. And just because you later move on in your career and find a new mentor, your contact doesn't have to end. My mentors, past and present, are some of my closest friends.

While I probably could have begun active research without a doctoral degree, I believed that I needed the credential to legitimize my existence in the male-dominated world of research. Once I had the degree, though, I gained experience quickly. Over the past two decades I have been involved with dozens of projects examining issues in African-American and Latino populations. In fact, I am now completing a study that has lasted for more than five years.

This study examined African Americans who had renal problems requiring hemodialysis. Specifically, we wanted to study the dynamics of how dialysis-dependent renal problems affected the patient and the family. Did the stress of chronic illness produce mental health problems for one or the other?

While we have not yet analyzed all the data, our preliminary findings are very interesting. Most patients had come to grips with their physical illness. The mere presence of disease did not compromise their mental health, but it appears that the manner in which the patient accepted treatment might. Some of our earlier work suggested that patients who complied with prescribed therapy seemed to deteriorate more quickly than those who did not. They were more likely to experience depression — and were more likely to die. Those who were less compliant experienced more positive outcomes. On the surface, this seems to contradict conventional medical thinking about the importance of compliance. However, we found that similar evidence had been uncovered in a small pilot study that took place nearly 10 years ago. We hypothesized that many patients who are compliant believe their condition is the beginning of the end of their lives. Their passivity and acceptance leads down a path to decline and death. Conversely, those who are less compliant are actually more interested and active in their own care. They are the fighters, the "difficult" patients who seek to know all they can about their disease. They listen to their body and recognize its cues, and they use that information to decide when treatment is needed. In other words, they set their own schedules, which may differ from the prescribed regimen. Instead of coming in three times a week, they may elect to come twice a week, or once a week. A patient after several treatments may decide some of the physicians and nurses working at the clinic aren't skilled at setting up and calibrating the dialysis machine. As a result, he may learn how to hook himself up to the machine and insist on doing so. Some of the clinic staff might think this person is a difficult patient, but I question that assumption. In fact, there is an old saying that the patient who has a prolonged illness may be his own best doctor. Hopefully, the data from our study will show that this may indeed be true. We may have to redefine what we call compliance and the way we listen to and interact with patients.

Some of our data on families suggest a link between the patient's condition and the mental health of the family members. Relatives who have extensive outside support groups and activities, including church groups and social clubs, had a far lower incidence of depression than those who lacked such connections. When depression occurred, it did so regardless of the patient's spirits or progress.

One of the primary features of a career in research is that it never gets boring. The questions answered by one study can spawn new considerations that demand exploration. For example, this project established more evidence for the positive results of noncompliance, opening the door for further research. And during our study of chronically ill patients and their relatives, we encountered families that had more than one relative on dialysis. This raises a number of new questions: Are these families more or less mentally stable than others? Does the mental and/or physical health of one patient affect the other? Is there something about the behavior, diet, genetics, or socioeconomic background of this family that led to such an incidence of diabetes? How does the death of a patient with a long-standing chronic illness affect the mental and physical health of surviving family members? The last question is the basis for a project we recently started — a $1.7 million study of bereavement's effects on surviving family members over a three-year period.

This brings up another important component of research: money. Despite the fact that billions of dollars are available for clinical research, funding is often difficult to find, especially for investigators who are unproven. The best way to establish a track record is with small pilot studies, short-term projects that pursue new lines of inquiry in small populations over a brief period of time. Pilot studies cost only a few thousand dollars, but they may generate data that can justify an expanded study.

No matter what the size of the study or how much money is needed to support it, the solution to funding lies in finding a source with compatible interests. Sometimes the source may have an entire list of criteria, but in other cases it is enough for a researcher to include only a statement of objectives. Funding is an area in which mentors can be very helpful to nurses who have limited research experience.

Nurses have one asset that is invaluable for a successful research career: clinical experience. In fact, I am convinced that nurses are better qualified to perform clinical research than many other health care professionals. Why? Because of their education and clinical experience. Accredited graduate courses for nurses involve learning the research process and actually participating in research projects. This is not required of physicians. Then, as nurses enter clinical practice, they learn to assess patients who present with a wide range of problems and to create care plans that focus on specific solutions. As a result, nurses develop skills in practical analysis, patient contact, assessment, interaction with other health care professionals, verbal and written communication, and following through. Other health professionals have to develop them along the way.

Research does not have to be clinical in nature. Indeed, many hospitals, HMOs, and other health care facilities use nurse-researchers to study issues in quality control, cost efficiency, and the effectiveness of care. But whatever area an investigator focuses on, the search will be for answers that lead to improved care for countless patients. It's a very special way of fulfilling nursing's mission.

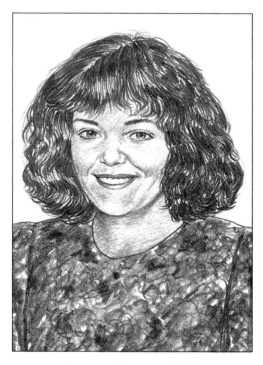

Suzanne Cavanaugh, RN,
is manager of clinical research administration
at Pfizer Pharmaceuticals,
New York, New York.

The Nurse in Industry

While most of my 19-year career has been in direct patient care or hospital administration, I have been working for the past five years in the pharmaceutical industry. My skills are fully utilized in this setting, and my work is so challenging that I'm constantly learning. I love it.

I initially attended a diploma program that was clinically and scientifically intensive. Although diploma programs are now virtually extinct, my education gave me a foundation of professional skills that have served me well.

After graduation, I worked for three years in a community hospital in a research-oriented unit. The unit was staffed with nine new graduates (three from each type of nursing training program: associate, diploma, baccalaureate) and was attempting to study the longevity of clinical careers in relation to education. Unit staff were also examining whether disruptive geriatric patients become more cooperative when they receive focused and goal-oriented nursing care.

This experience, along with my education, gave me a solid medical-surgical background, but I began to feel the need for more focus in my career.

I had enjoyed my psych rotation in school, so I took a position as a staff nurse in a psychiatric hospital. I made a two-year commitment to work there, but I stayed for 11 years.

The unit was involved in groundbreaking research in the diagnosis and treatment of intractable, borderline character-disordered patients. It was a long-term care unit, and I was among the first group of nurses hired to staff it. Because the unit was new, we had to sift through a population of mostly psychotic patients in order to identify a character-disordered population. This took about 18 months, and while the environment was chaotic, it was diagnostically diversified and gave me a broad base of knowledge. Just as the unit was becoming cohesive, I was offered an administrative position that put me in charge of the day shift and required that I serve as a liaison between the nursing staff (composed of RNs and mental health workers) and the nursing care coordinator and her assistant. I was also team leader for a specific group of long-term patients, and this entailed weekly decision-making sessions with patients and the nursing staff to determine how much responsibility and freedom the patients were able to assume. In dealing with this population, which is known for episodes of intense rage, I learned a lot about myself, about professionalism, and about nuances of human behavior. Also, I was at the center of decision making for nursing policy and structuring of the milieu, which emphasized patient participation and responsibility — and safety, too, since many of these patients were suicidal.

I held that position for about five years. Then, the unit underwent a generational change, and many of the original staff, including the unit chief and nursing care coordinator, left. I applied for and obtained the nursing care coordinator position, which increased my administrative and clinical skills. I began to feel professionally mature. I had almost complete responsibility for the structure of the inpatient milieu and for the nursing care given on this unit. I became more involved in off-unit administrative committees and decision-making bodies as well.

As nursing care coordinator, I covered occasional weekends for the nursing supervisors, and this added to my community experience, mostly in handling emergency admissions and manning the suicide hotline.

The 14 years of nursing experience described here gave me a solid background in direct clinical care and administration as well as a familiarity with research. After working solely in hospitals, mostly with seriously ill patients, I was having a career crisis: I wanted a major change.

I knew two people who were working for Pfizer Pharmaceuticals, and both encouraged me to apply there. I was doubtful about making such a drastic switch, but decided that at least I could use the opportunity to further assess my professional abilities in an environment where I had less direct responsibility for other people, and to see where I wanted to go from there.

Well, that was five years ago, and pharmaceuticals has become a wonderful new career for me. I joined Pfizer as a consultant clinical research associate (CRA) and currently am manager of research administration for anti-infectives in a marketing division.

The clinical research associate position is a great starting point for a nurse. The structure of the job requires dual responsibilities: those of a team member in the research and marketing of a given product, and those of a professional in carrying out the job in compliance with regulations established by internal corporate policy and the Food and Drug Administration.

FDA regulations are key to much of a clinical research associate's job, and nursing experience is extremely helpful, because we have already been trained to be aware of legal and regulatory issues and to weave them into the job at hand.

A CRA is usually assigned to work on a particular pharmaceutical product. As a member of a medical team, this person monitors research that produces data to support our knowledge about a drug and provide the marketing and sales division with specific scientific information that helps establish the drug as an integral part of health care planning in the community.

For these studies to be carried out in a consistent fashion and within FDA regulations, someone must be administratively responsible for the paperwork, finances, and monitoring of actual case entries. This person is the CRA.

For instance, a pharmaceutical company physician and a community physician will discuss a potential clinical study utilizing a particular product. The study is put into a format called a protocol, which outlines the scientific premise of the study and specific methods of gathering and formulating data.

After the basic protocol has been formulated, a CRA is assigned to finalize its details with consistent input from medical, statistical, and regulatory personnel. In addition, the CRA must assure that required documents are filed at Pfizer and the study site, that supplies, including the drug itself, are ordered for the site, and that documents verify the fully informed consent of all patients and the accredited licensure of study personnel.

At the beginning of a study, a case report form must be devised. This is a tool for documenting study information on site, and it should be clear and comprehensive. The format should enable data entry and, ultimately, analysis. While all of this may sound routine, I appreciated my earlier experience when I began this job, because I was immediately assigned to work on 30 studies in different phases. I had to jump in and quickly learn how to prioritize accurately in juggling all of this work. There was minimal orientation, but I was fortunate enough to be working with highly qualified professionals who helped me adjust without making terrible errors.

Another aspect of this job is on-site monitoring, which can be enjoyable as well as critical to the work. It requires traveling (for me, within the continental United States) to assess the progress of studies. Each case entered must be reviewed page by page, checked against the medical record to verify accuracy, and assessed for eligibility on the basis of protocol criteria. While much of this is straightforward, much is not, because many clinical cases have gray areas, study site personnel have varying levels of expertise, and cooperation can be limited. So I may, for example, get involved in lengthy discussions with the site coordinator, who often is a nurse, and/or the investigator (the MD/PhD responsible for the study) regarding enrollment of complicated patients, scientific and clinical definition of outcomes, study parameters, and failures of documentation. Particularly critical is the assessment of adverse reactions and insuring that these are reported quickly and accurately. Because these discussions can be difficult at times, diplomacy and clinical knowledge are both valuable assets. While some interactions are difficult, it's generally fun to be in a nice city like San Francisco or Chicago or, possibly, a quiet farm town in Idaho, and to interact with professionals who are dedicated to learning and advancing knowledge about patient care, research, and pharmaceutical agents.

Above and beyond individual study activity are the ever-present and, for me, fascinating dynamics of how and why a system works, and what I can do to be involved administratively. I guess my previous experience conditioned me to get significantly involved from the beginning at Pfizer, even though the industry details were new to me at the time. Thanks to my nursing skills, I am able to organize, prioritize, deal with stress and crisis, and interact with a myriad of managers, peers, and subordinates.

Because of this experience and some turnover during my first few years here, I am once again in a supervisory position. This industry is challenging in terms of regulation, politics, community interaction, and many other aspects. For me, the main difference between a hospital and an industry setting is intensity. Here, even though the responsibilities are great, the life-and-death pressures of a hospital do not exist. And yet, I'm dealing with important health care issues that keep me focused and present me with continuing challenge. In fact, my work takes place on the cutting edge of all sorts of scientific research and technology. When we make an important discovery, my efforts have contributed to the health of not just one patient, but thousands. I'm still very much in the health care arena, and my goal is still to deliver quality care to patients.

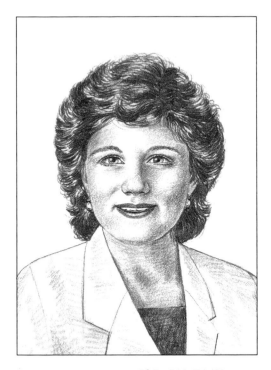

Patricia Moccia, PhD, RN, FAAN,
is chief operating officer and
executive vice president of
the National League for Nursing,
New York, New York.

Opportunity in a Professional Association

As a social-minded teenager in the middle 1960s, I wanted to go south on the freedom bus rides. Not surprisingly, my mother didn't think that was a good idea. She convinced me that I could help people more directly by staying in New York and volunteering in a hospital. I worked first as a candystriper, then as an aide, and my experiences there made my career choice plain: I wanted to be a nurse.

I was all set to enter a diploma program, but my head nurse recommended I choose a baccalaureate program instead. I looked into the New York University five-year program, and adolescent logic told me that if four years were better than three, then five were better than four. I enrolled.

My undergraduate years took place in an era of social revolution. I joined the student nurse association and actively protested against what was going on in Southeast Asia. Throughout my college years, I stayed involved in social issues, demonstrating a dedication that eventually led to my current job as chief operating officer and executive vice president of the National League for Nursing.

I've always felt that a nurse's work—and the work of health care professionals in general—is a particular manifestation of the larger goal of effecting social change. Fortunately, my baccalaureate education emphasized the philosophy of community-based nursing—that nursing takes place where the people are. In my work, I felt it was incumbent on me to help people understand how larger social issues affect their health.

After earning my BSN, I attended graduate school for a semester, then left feeling that the program didn't give me the opportunity I wanted to engage with the community. I discovered that I didn't like feeling removed from the issues of the day and that my energies were not being used to make a difference in people's lives.

So, to exercise my philosophy that health care workers should work directly with the community, and because I was interested in psychology, I withdrew from school and became absorbed by community health issues, focusing my energy on the deinstitutionalization of the mentally ill. We worked with patients at a Boston hospital and moved them into community settings, developing home care programs and clinics staffed by lay workers. I stayed there two years, then returned to school. In 1975, I graduated with a master's in systems theory, which focused on psychology and holistic nursing. In 1980, I was awarded my doctorate. My dissertation philosophically investigated the relationship between theory and practice. I studied the dynamic between the whole and the parts, focusing on what nurses needed to do idealistically and practically to achieve a holistic practice.

After completing my doctorate, I had a decision-making crisis: I didn't know whether I wanted to remain in academia. As a result, I took a leave of absence to join a project in Appalachia that was sponsored by the U.S. Public Health Service and the American Lung Association. There I helped establish clinics to work with the families of miners with black-lung disease. In addition to the clinical aspects of this job, I found myself troubled by the fact that this disease could be prevented by better working conditions. That experience sparked an interest in occupational health, and I did postdoctoral work at the University of Cincinnati, setting up occupational health programs at Hunter College in New York.

Over this time there was a definite evolution in my interests, but the underlying theory that illness can be socially manufactured or perpetuated remained intact. I continued the relationship I had started as an undergraduate with the health policy advisory center, and I published papers on social and economic factors that contribute to disease, including why women's diseases were not well researched and why black populations have less access to the health system than they need. I became the chair of nursing education programs at Columbia University's teacher's college. In that capacity, I worked in graduate programs, teaching nurses who wanted to become faculty or administrators of nursing services. We had wonderful seminars on bringing theory and practice together and on ways nursing can be used to change society. We discussed new ways of developing curricula and teaching students, and the program became very socially active.

Then came the catch. We were doing exciting things, but the nurses, who loved the ideas, found that the accrediting committee of the National League for Nursing (NLN) wouldn't allow them to be implemented. The NLN's stringent accreditation criteria generally didn't encourage much interaction between nursing academia and the community. Once again, I had collided with the ivory tower.

However, within the league was a group of people who were advocates of curriculum revolution. These nurses were calling for changes that would result in nonhierarchical student-teacher relationships, as well as increased involvement in communities. In general, there was a sense among the membership that the time for reform had come.

Change was in the air, and the timing proved auspicious for me. I was known through my writing and soon became involved in this issue. In 1988, I joined the NLN as vice president for accreditation. I was responsible for reviewing all accreditation policies and working with the membership to discuss policies it wanted changed. I increased the number of people involved in policy evaluation and started a move to define outcome criteria and increase public accountability for programs. What did we expect of our graduates? Once we could answer that question definitively, we would be able to employ greater flexibility in achieving our expectations. Our definition of education became broader, and we worked with the league's faculty and practicing members to increase their involvement with each other.

In the past, members would call and ask can we do this? Often, the league would answer no, you can't; you won't be accredited. As we were able to change our internal philosophy, the answer increasingly became yes, you can.

In 1990, I became executive vice president of the NLN, adding to my responsibilities those of coordinating other NLN activities, including test design, research, and communications through books and videos. At meetings and seminars, I report on resources members need in order to be well served in their jobs, and I work with the divisions to develop programs that can address those needs. I rely heavily on my staff — recruited in the membership division — to report back to me from the front lines.

About one half of our membership hails from academia, one quarter comes from practicing nurses in acute care and community health settings, and the rest comes from nurses in such specialty fields as informatics or research. Currently, I am trying to develop a network that will bring these nurses together to reflect our common nursing interests and values. Also, we want to expand our membership to incorporate students, nurse practitioners, and those in other segments of the profession.

Within the league, I help decide where nursing should be going. If we're deciding whether to develop a certain kind of test or program, our priorities now are on community health and primary care, as well as the importance of developing strategies that reflect new ways of thinking about acute care. As the pendulum swings away from the financially intensive needs of acute care to the cost-effective arena of primary care, we're trying to attract resources to support that shift while facilitating the efforts of nurses in that field. For instance, we work with lobbyists to change legal and regulatory restrictions that prevent nurses from writing prescriptions or having hospital admitting privileges.

I'm on the road two or three days a week, talking with members and representing the NLN to other nursing and professional organizations. I meet with constituent leagues and report what I hear from them in newsletters and journals. While I don't hold a teaching faculty position, I frequently give guest lectures, and I serve as an adviser on an occasional doctoral project.

Over and over, members tell me that the NLN needs to address the changing student and patient populations. We must adapt nursing education and practices to reflect the diversities of age, race, and ethnicity, because the minorities that used to exist are quickly becoming majorities. In the area of education, the age of nurses entering school is rising rapidly. They're not all coming straight out of high school, either. In fact, nursing may not be their first career. They may be raising families. All of these factors call for flexible thinking in academia.

Today, some of our members have formed coalitions among community groups, schools, and homeless shelters to bring a nursing perspective and expertise to the impact social issues have on people's health. Of course, I am proud of this because it echoes back to my roots in community activism and my desire to view nursing as one part in the greater whole of social structure. This philosophy is even reflected in our name: We're the National League for Nursing, not the National League of Nurses.

It's imperative that I keep up with the politics surrounding health care, because I am leading the organization at a critical juncture. As the Clinton administration seeks to revamp the health care system, I have tried to make the NLN as available and influential as possible. Happily, we have more access to policy makers than ever before. Indeed, many of our members have been asked to develop background papers and serve on task forces. As I meet with representatives from the AMA and health insurers, I feel like I've died and gone to heaven just to be talking about health care reform. We may not always be talking the same community-based health care language, but at least we're talking.

I'm well aware that philosophically and pragmatically I am standing on the shoulders of the people who came before me in this organization. Still, whoever holds this job must be a visionary. I see my role — and I've trained my staff to see theirs — as one of executing the decisions of our membership. We gather information, gauge the feelings of the membership, and make recommendations about ways to focus their activities but, ultimately, the membership decides what to do. Of course, the membership's priorities may not always coincide with mine, yet that doesn't frustrate me. I know that our basic values are in synchronization. I simply take the attitude that there are a million things to do in this world, and at least I'm getting some of them done.

To enjoy a career in a professional organization, I think the most important thing is to be committed to a process rather than an outcome. My own commitment is to the idea of nurses and other health care professionals working together. If you have a specific idea of what nursing should do next, you would probably be happier serving in an elected position. But as a staff member, I must focus on helping my colleagues achieve those specific goals. The difference is between working for a special interest or furthering the overall interests of the membership.

The second thing in considering a career in a nursing association is that nursing is a business. We deal with corporations, not with people just sitting around talking about how to help each other. Still, we are a socially conscious business, and I strive to have the NLN demonstrate in its operation the same qualities we think are important in society. Here, you need a vision of what health care can be, what nurses can do, and how 150 staff members can work together. This is a high-pressure job. To do it well requires considerable maturity.

That it is worth doing is clear, because nursing and health care must be seen in the context of a larger society. Now, more than ever before, nurses who work in associations have an opportunity to shape the future of health care in America.

The VA Nurse

Frankie T. Manning, MA, RN,
is chief of nursing services at the
Seattle VA Medical Center.

Growing up in a small Texas town, I quickly learned who were the most important people in the community: the doctor, the nurse, and the mortician. My first career aspiration was to be a mortician, but the field didn't offer much opportunity for a black female. Medical school was out of the question because we couldn't afford it. My great-aunt was a midwife, and I knew she was respected, because all the white people called her "Miss Sarah." She was able to cross over the race barrier by virtue of what she did for a living. So I decided to enter nursing.

In 1957, I earned my diploma from St. John's School of Nursing in Tulsa, Okla. My first job offer was to teach at St. John's School of Nursing, but the offer was withdrawn when the administration began to worry that hiring me as the first black teacher would cause problems. I didn't want to be anywhere people didn't want me, so I went to work as a staff nurse in the black ward of St. John's Hospital. I stayed there until 1962, worked at a Delaware hospital for a year, then in 1963 went to Japan as a Red Cross nurse. When I returned to the United States in 1966, I started working for the Department of Veterans Affairs (VA) in Wichita, Kan. That was my professional introduction to the agency I still work for—now as chief of nursing services at the Seattle VA Medical Center (VAMC).

Actually, my first contact with the VA was during my high school days, when I used to sing for patients at a VA medical center. I thought of the VA as an old folks' home and, to be honest, I wasn't particularly excited about working there because I was more interested in acute care. So when I started as a staff nurse at the 300-bed facility, I was surprised to find that the focus was on acute care. I worked in orthopedics, critical care, and the recovery room, dealing with an interesting mix of patients. There were many World War II veterans, but that was at the height of the Vietnam conflict, and many severely injured young men were coming back.

I didn't understand why Americans were so against veterans. I was married to a Vietnam vet, and I certainly didn't have the impression that these men were hippies on drugs. Interestingly, I never saw animosity between my World War II patients and my Vietnam war patients. Instead, the older vets acted as surrogate fathers and were committed to helping these kids.

I learned some important lessons about nursing care there. In particular, I remember one young man, about 24, who had multiple abdominal wounds and legs so badly injured he would never walk again. He was extremely angry about his injuries and spent a lot of time making everybody miserable. As we began to work with him, we discovered he had some ideas about his own care. As nurses, we thought we knew best, and that was where the conflict arose. At times he became so infuriated about not being allowed to influence the way we cared for him that he wouldn't let anyone touch him. Obviously we needed some sort of compromise. So, we began to give him a few of the things he wanted: We let him help change his own dressings, and we let him have a beer in the evening. That last request was not unreasonable, but the prevailing belief that these men were alcoholics and dopeheads made many nurses think alcohol was inappropriate in the hospital.

Another touchy issue involved visits from his girlfriend. While he had no movement below the waist, this didn't prevent him from relating to her sexually, and some of the nurses had fits just knowing what was going on. But, after making sure the woman was aware of basic safety issues — such as making sure the patient didn't fall out of bed — we let them visit privately. As we allowed him to participate and exercise some control over his life, we saved a great deal of time, because he wasn't resisting every step of the way.

VA nurses deal primarily with men and must be mindful of the fact that there is a certain sense of machismo, control, and power to cope with. However, I've found that our patients are more compliant than in a general hospital. They're used to taking orders, and if you tell them to go to the bathroom at eight, 10, and 12 o'clock, they will. It's a question of balancing their need to feel in control.

I stayed at the Wichita VA Hospital until 1974. In that same year, I received my BSN from Wichita State University School of Nursing. I stayed on at the school for a year to teach community health and beginning medical-surgical nursing. After that, I went to the VA Hospital in Iowa City as assistant chief nurse. This is a large research-oriented hospital close to the University of Iowa, so my clinical responsibilities were skewed toward academic health care. There I developed clinical programs, including one that expanded the number of levels in critical and acute care, and one that made it possible for us to see outpatients in a more timely fashion.

I stayed in Iowa City from 1976 to 1978, during which time I completed my master's in nursing administration with a medical-surgical minor from the University of Iowa. I worked at the Portland VAMC from 1978 until 1980, then came to the Seattle VAMC in 1981 as chief nurse.

Seattle VAMC is a 428-bed acute medical-surgical facility with a 60-bed nursing home. It was here that the prosthetic Seattle Foot was created, and we've just installed a new computer system that helps ensure a better fit for artificial limbs. We've had great success with double amputees. In addition, we have programs in alcohol and substance abuse, acute psychiatry, and posttraumatic stress disorder (PTSD), all of which are common among VAMC patients.

As chief of nursing services, I oversee all clinical aspects of care, manage staff, and serve as an adviser to the hospital on patient care issues. As a result, I look at things from the hospital level as well as the nursing level. For instance, I'm currently chairing a hospital-wide task force that is considering how to improve the admissions process. I'm involved in community and university activities as they relate to health care, and I work with national committees within the VA including the search committee that is looking for an assistant chief medical director for nursing programs. At the community level, I'm working with the local cancer society and the United Way to find ways these two groups can work together to improve the quality of cancer care.

With 172 hospitals, the VA is the largest organized health care system in the world, and we have the largest nursing service. Thus, one distinct advantage of working in the VA is the chance nurses have to network within the system. If I have a problem in Seattle, I have access to 171 other chief nurses who can advise me and tell me what they've done in similar cases. My staff has the same option. In essence, we have a built-in and free consultant service. At Seattle VAMC, we have two experts in diabetes, and people call them from all over for advice on related issues. This network was invaluable when the country was experiencing the height of the nursing shortage in the mid-1980s. Our computer lines were quite busy as chief nurses and nurse recruiters were trying to figure out how to recruit and retain nurses.

I rarely get involved directly with clinical responsibilities, but it does happen. Recently, we were short-staffed, so I worked nights in our nursing home. I scored big points with my staff, and I loved renewing my connection with bedside nursing. There's nothing better than having a patient say, "You really made me feel better."

But most of my day is spent in meetings and taking care of administrative issues. During a recent day, I met with a task force at 7:30 AM, then with a consultant to review data analysis for a new computer program. I made several telephone calls and then had a meeting with a staff member who has a history of substance abuse. After that, I met with a community group to explore ways we might build a consortium to provide care to geriatric clients, and then I came back to meet with my executive staff about staff distribution and major problem areas in nursing service. In addition, I spend time precepting nursing administration students and providing management development training for my staff.

A major difference between a VA chief of nursing services and a nurse with the same title in a private setting is that I have less money to work with. Also, my colleagues in the private world often have jurisdiction over supporting departments, such as respiratory, dietary, and social work — I don't. I'm working to change things so that those areas will report to nursing, but until that happens, my job is a little harder because I find that I am constantly negotiating with those departments.

VA medical care has not always had the best reputation, but I think most of that is due to a misunderstanding on the part of the public. Certainly there's no question that we in the VA have made mistakes. Still, after having worked in other hospitals, I believe the VA is the best system I can imagine for providing continuity of care. We're a major national asset. In fact, I believe we're second only to the NIH in research.

As is true throughout health care, the VA is working to provide more outpatient and community-based care. We're also adjusting to the fact that we're seeing female patients in increasing numbers. Most VA nurses have dealt primarily with men, but now we're having to learn a whole new system that focuses on women's issues. In the past five years, most of my staff have been trained to understand the physiological differences, and we have systems in place that will help us deal with women in a comprehensive, rather than an ad hoc, manner. For instance, we contract with a gynecologist for her services, and I have a nurse practitioner who deals solely with women's reproductive issues.

When I hire nurses, I look for someone who's absolutely committed to caring for patients from birth to death, because that's the nature of the VA patient. I need nurses who have a strong sense of community but, because many of our patients come to us from long distances — Alaska, Idaho, Montana — they have to be able to follow up beyond the community. A sense of family is crucial, too. We deal with a lot of older men, and although their wives are not veterans, they need care just as much as their husbands. And, because we employ our own physicians, VA nurses have greater control over the patients' care, so they need good problem-solving skills.

The VA system offers the broadest imaginable spectrum of care — from prescription eyeglasses to liver transplants — and our nurses can transfer from one VA hospital to another without loss of benefits. Each hospital has its own areas of excellence and opportunities for academic collaboration or research. A nurse who wants career flexibility but doesn't want to start over at ground zero with every move would be hard-pressed to find a better place to work. Personally, I love watching nurses develop. It is surprising how quickly they reach the stage where they come into my office not with problems, but with solutions.

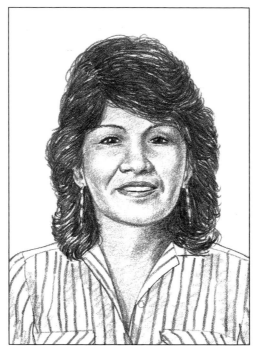

Sally N. Pete, MSN, RN,
is a public health nursing program
coordinator for the Indian Health Service,
Winslow, Arizona.

Nursing in the Indian Health Service

Viruses, germs, and *microscopes* have at least one thing in common: They are English words that do not translate into the Navajo language.

One aspect of my job as a public health nursing program coordinator with the Indian Health Service is explaining western medical technologies in terms that are understandable to Navajo people who speak no English. I'm a full-blooded Navajo, and I speak both Navajo and English. My job is to bring western medicine to a traditional Indian culture. I'm based in Winslow, Ariz., where I'm the health coordinator for about 3,000 Navajo Indians who live on the reservation. I joined the Indian Health Service because I wanted to stay close to my family and the reservation. In fact, even though I'm living in Winslow, my permanent home is on the reservation.

As a community health nurse, I have worked in the field with Hopi and Navajo tribes, providing such basic health services as immunizations and screening for vision and hearing, and following up with patients who had been recently discharged from the hospital. When we visited patients who lived in remote areas, we often were accompanied by a physician. Otherwise, our care was based on protocols set by physicians.

Pneumonia, obesity, diabetes, diarrhea, and dehydration are common problems in Native American populations. In addition, we saw women who needed prenatal or postpartum care, as well as older people who had pneumonia, cardiac problems, or diabetes, which is particularly common among Hopi patients.

The Navajo used to be a very active people, busily engaged in such day-to-day chores as herding sheep and hauling wood and water. But that has changed and now they live more sedentary lives. I believe that is why there is a preponderance of medical problems (eg, diabetes, cardiac disease, and hypertension) that are related to a lack of physical exercise.

It is very difficult to get patients — especially older ones — to make basic lifestyle changes. You can urge them to get more exercise, to cut back on fats, and to include more fruits and vegetables in their diets, but their compliance usually is frustratingly low. It takes constant reinforcement for people to begin changing. Sometimes, though, something drastic happens to make a person realize what's at stake. I remember one man who had a heart attack and required bypass surgery. Afterwards, he began eating more intelligently. He nagged his children about their diets and, because they had seen the way he suffered, they began living more healthy lives.

I'm seeing more pregnancy among teenagers than ever before. I also believe alcoholism and substance abuse are increasing, and as a direct consequence, so is domestic violence, as well as child abuse and neglect. Nevertheless, some of the problems that plague the general U.S. population are less prevalent in the Navajo population. For one thing, we don't see as many drug-affected babies. Also, Navajos — especially women — rarely smoke, although there's a high use of smokeless tobacco.

I helped set up a program in a tribal jail to which nurses came once or twice a week to treat inmates and refer them to hospitals as needed. I also worked with our staff pediatrics nurse practitioner to establish a well-child clinic. We made home visits to all newborns to make sure everything was going well. Sometimes we ran into cases of suspected child abuse or neglect, and we would refer these to social services or other appropriate resources.

This close involvement in case management is a big part of nursing care in the Indian Health Service; I spend much of my time coordinating services with physicians and social services, including mental health and alcohol treatment programs. That's a major advantage in the Indian Health Service: There's always somewhere to turn for assistance. In the private sector, especially for low-income minority populations, the only option may be a financially strapped and inadequate county system. Here, there are always resources to which we can refer.

I recently earned my master's degree, with a focus on administration in community health nursing. Working on my degree, I did an analysis of Navajo perceptions of the word *harmony,* particularly as it relates to health. That project has proven to be very useful as I now try to balance modern medical care with traditional Navajo values. The Navajo integrate religious and spiritual beliefs and ideas of health into an overall concept of well-being. They believe that man should live in harmony with all earthly things — including other humans, plants, rain, thunder — and that, as long as he does not harm anything, he will always remain healthy. If he violates those principles and enters a state of disharmony, he will experience hardship or sickness.

As a result of this, older people in particular, and some younger ones who have been raised in the old way, may feel guilty if they get sick; they think they've done something wrong. In such cases, it can be difficult to explain that a patient's diarrhea is the consequence of what the person ate, not something he or she *did.* In this area, the ability to provide effective health education is a critical part of the job.

When working with Native Americans, you must never lose sight of the fact that a completely different set of values and beliefs will have an influence on the delivery of health care. It is not at all uncommon, for example, for patients to visit a tribal medicine man before going to a hospital. I believe it is essential to respect that desire, because if it helps a patient psychologically and spiritually, it is likely to help physically and promote the healing process. Besides, medicine men employ some practices (especially herbal remedies) that have proven effective over the years. Still, if a medicine man knows he can't help, he will suggest that the person try modern medicine. By the same token, in some situations — say when a person is grieving — I might suggest he seek the medicine man's counsel.

At times, a combination of modern and traditional approaches can be useful. For instance, if a Navajo falls and breaks his ankle, he might make use of the modern health care system by having it set and cast. He also might visit the medicine man, who probably would suggest that giving a sacrament to the earth would help the patient feel absolved spiritually.

Those at the headquarters of the Indian Health Service have certain goals they want to achieve by the year 2000. Part of my job is to implement those goals at a local level. As an example of this, we are maintaining our 90-percent immunization rate, but we are also in the process of reorganizing our immunization program to focus on children under 27 months of age. These children have immunization cards and computer records, so we are able to see what immunizations they have been given and which ones they're missing. Using these records, we develop a deficiency list that we send to our public health nurses so they can contact patients directly. At the same time, we're trying to teach people to assume greater responsibility for their own health care. We encourage them to visit the clinic for their immunizations instead of waiting for us to go to them. Reducing the incidence of teen pregnancy is another IHS priority, and we're trying to do this through health promotion programs in schools.

I'm working to address the needs of high-risk and underserved patient populations — mostly children and the elderly — who could easily slip through the cracks in our health care system unless someone goes out of the way for them. In this category is a diabetic woman who kept missing her appointments because of other problems, including alcohol abuse and family problems. She spoke only Navajo, and her family had more or less stopped trying to help her. Clearly, this woman needed extra attention, so I made a special effort to go out and talk with her about the importance of managing her diabetes.

I'm indirectly responsible for about 3,000 patients, a huge case load that is manageable only with the help of nurses' aides and other community health representatives who serve as liaisons to our office. Actually, I spend only half my time on the reservation providing in-home patient care to between 20 and 25 patients a week. When I am in the office, I review immunization records and coordinate with the field workers to help children who have special problems. I spend a large part of my time planning health education programs for schools because the IHS is beginning to increase its emphasis on health promotion and disease prevention.

A person who wants a career working with Native Americans needs the strongest possible clinical background. While it's not necessary to be a Native American, it is necessary to understand the Indian culture and the special circumstances in which ethnic minorities live. For this reason, courses in anthropology or sociology will be valuable. The liberal arts education achieved in a baccalaureate program is so important that the Indian Health Service now requires that all public health nurses have a BSN.

The years I have spent in the Indian Health Service have been great. I've been able to advance my education in a way that I probably could not otherwise have afforded. As a result, I have developed skills that make it possible for me to help people who really need it and, in fact, whose lives might be diminished without it. When I go out in the field, it feels like going home.

(The opinions expressed in this article are those of the author and do not necessarily reflect the views of the Indian Health Service.)

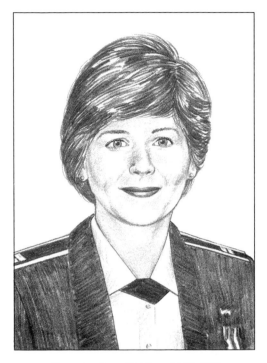

Captain Cary Collins, BSN, RN,
is a nurse recruitment supervisor
at McGuire AFB, New Jersey.

The Air Force Nurse

When people ask me why I joined the Air Force, my glib answer is "I like jets." Certainly, the excitement and thrill of serving in the Air Force was part of my decision, but there's a lot more, too.

After earning my BSN in 1977, I became a surgical staff nurse at a hospital near my New Jersey home. Three years later, I felt that I had learned all I was going to learn there, and I was growing impatient for a change in my life. In retrospect, I think it was then that the idea of joining the Air Force lodged in the back of my mind.

I left the hospital and spent another three years providing home care with the visiting nurse association. By the end of that period, I still wasn't satisfied. I couldn't put my finger on it, but I felt that something was missing. I started to think long-term, about going back to school and even about a complete change of careers. But first, I decided to investigate the Air Force. I liked what I saw, and in 1984 I signed up as a psychiatric nurse. I spent the next seven years working on mental health units. Now I'm on a special duty assignment as chief of the nurse recruiting branch at McGuire Air Force Base in New Jersey.

Nursing in the Air Force differs somewhat from a civilian setting in that Air Force nurses have medical technicians working with them. These technicians can start IVs and draw blood, freeing the nurses to perform more baccalaureate-oriented duties, including teaching, assessment, intervention, care planning, and working with families.

I began psychiatric nursing in a large teaching hospital on an Air Force base. The psychiatric unit was organized into an independent community with its own constitution and president. Patients voted on such issues as whether to increase or diminish the privileges available to individuals on the ward. The nurses monitored the community and acted as catalysts, encouraging the patients to work together and help themselves. In addition, we kept charts, administered medications, and supervised technicians. Working with a psychologist, we helped run group therapy sessions and assessed the response of patients — whether they were overstimulated or being given more responsibility than they could handle. Part of the job was to be aware if patients were hallucinating or beginning to withdraw, and to know which ones needed more aggressive care.

In short, I was an essential part of the team, and physicians depended on me for my professional judgement.

Occasionally we saw cases of posttraumatic stress disorder. Interestingly, although that's commonly associated with war, we found a number of young women who suffered from this disorder as a result of sexual abuse in their childhood.

After four years in that assignment, I spent another four years stationed at a mental health unit in England.

While the types of diseases or injuries Air Force nurses see are similar to those seen in the civilian population, there are some differences in patients' health and attitudes. For example, Air Force patients, like military patients in general, are healthier than civilians. They're well nourished, physically fit, and tend to be drug free and HIV negative. Many of the underlying conditions that civilian nurses confront are infrequently seen in the military. I've found that patients are more polite and have a far higher rate of compliance. A likely reason for this is that our physicians and nurses are officers, and if they tell a patient to take his medicine, the patient obeys, because in the Air Force, a doctor's order is just that — an order.

In my current job, I oversee five recruiters who go to colleges and job fairs to present a program describing nursing opportunities in the Air Force. In addition to BSNs, we're looking for nurse practitioners, a growing field in the Air Force. We talk to nurse midwives, pediatrics nurse practitioners, nurse anesthetists, and OB/GYN practitioners about joining the Air Force.

As a supervisor, my primary job is to act as a nurse consultant. I tell prospective recruits what they can expect in an Air Force career, and I teach my recruiters what nurses do and how nurses think. In addition, I help them design programs that will be appropriate for a particular audience. I talk about the travel and camaraderie that characterize life in the military. If I'm talking to practicing nurses, I focus more on continuing education in the service and about the life and autonomy nursing officers can expect. Above all else, I emphasize the strong sense of professionalism among Air Force nurses. Nurses are officers, and their responsibilities and opportunities for recognition are greater than they would be in a civilian situation. Because we work as colleagues with physicians, the doctor-nurse relationship is also that of officer-to-officer. This increases the respect accorded nurses.

The other part of my job is to interview nurses, looking for leadership skills and the ability to adjust to change, and to recommend candidates to recruitment headquarters. Nurses we recruit must be able to handle the stress of moving away from familiar aspects of home and civilian life. They also must be able to apply common sense in meeting challenges they weren't exposed to in school.

I believe the Air Force has very high standards. Nurses we accept have the highest test scores, and we require our nurses to have a BSN.

Nurses who are specialists may enter the Air Force with the expectation of practicing in that specialty. Everyone else comes in as a bedside nurse. Some nurses are drawn to the military hoping for a job in management or such high-profile areas as the ER or ICU. Most Air Force nurses begin as staff nurses and move up.

After joining the Air Force, nurses go through an intensive 16-day officers' training program. Then, they are assigned to bedside duties. A nurse could continue indefinitely in the clinical role, but after several years some select a career path as a beginning manager. Many of our nurses have opportunities to return to school for a master's degree or consider specialty assignments in areas such as flight nursing or infection control.

In their third tours, after a total of four years in the service, most Air Force nurses become charge nurses and assume duties in clinical coordination, management, or teaching. They might apply for special duty assignments like mine, but to do that they should have gone through two rotations — one of them overseas, preferably.

All this time, the nurse will be moving up in rank. Most enter the service as second lieutenants. Two years later, they can expect a promotion to first lieutenant and in two more years to captain. Then they're in line to become majors.

One aspect of nursing that's specific to the Air Force is flight nursing. For that, nurses must attend flight school for five and a half weeks to learn about the physiology of flight — how altitude affects basic body systems. Another specialty open to Air Force nurses is hyperbaric nursing, which takes place in a chamber that can be pressurized with different gases and is used to treat dive illnesses as well as burns and other difficult-to-heal wounds. Some Air Force nurses work in air transportable hospitals that are deployed anywhere in support of fighting troops.

Unusual nursing opportunities aside, one of the strongest benefits of an Air Force career is that it gives nurses an unparalleled opportunity to exercise leadership and to change jobs frequently without sacrificing seniority. For instance, in the job I now have, I'm gaining experience in management, writing, and public speaking, while maintaining my rank. In a civilian position, it is far more difficult to change jobs. The military encourages it, and this goes a long way toward preventing burnout.

A full array of benefits is another compelling feature of life in the Air Force. Many of our nurses enter simply for the education benefits. Apart from educational support, we receive travel and shopping discounts as well as full medical benefits. Although salaries for military nurses initially are lower than might be seen in equivalent civilian positions, we receive longevity raises every two years and with every promotion in rank. Within three or four years, our earnings surpass those of our civilian counterparts. Our base pay is taxable income, but the food and housing allowances are not.

While I still say I'm taking the Air Force assignment to assignment, in the back of my mind I have a feeling I will be with the Air Force until I retire. After all, I have found the professionalism and the sense of purpose I was looking for as a civilian nurse. Besides, I still like those planes.

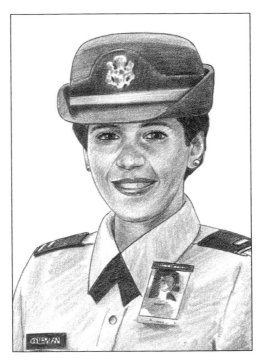

First Lieutenant Leonetta Coleman, BSN, RN,
is a surgical nurse at
Fitzsimons Army Medical Center in
Aurora, Colorado.

The Army Nurse

As an Army nurse, I have two careers — as a professional nurse and as an officer in the United States Army. This is a challenging blend of duties that gives me all the responsibility, and all the opportunity, I want. It is not always easy but, for me, the rewards have been outstanding.

I decided to become an Army nurse while I was in nursing school. I knew I wanted to practice in a hospital, but many of the nurses I met during training didn't seem as fulfilled as I thought they should have been. All too often, nurses were working in stressful, understaffed situations. To my mind, these conditions made it difficult to deliver ideal nursing care. And, strained work schedules left little time for the development of collaborative relationships between nurses and physicians. I had heard that life was different for Army nurses.

But the most important reason for my choosing this direction is that I am ambitious by nature and plan to seek advancement beyond a bedside staff position. Civilian hospital nurses whom I knew advanced slowly along their career paths. They needed years of experience before they could move into more specialized practices, and even more years there before they could assume supervisory roles. I always believed that advancement should be based on the capabilities of the individual rather than the predicted performance of the so-called average person. As a result, I began looking for other options and decided to learn more about the armed services. As it turned out, the Army was exactly what I wanted.

I accepted what is called a direct commission and, essentially, went straight from nursing school into the Army. I was offered a chance to defer my assignment, but I was anxious to get started in my practice. I chose the Army over other service branches because its program guaranteed that I would be able to obtain training in the specialty area of my choice — OB/GYN. Besides, my father had been in the Army and had always sung its praises. I figured if I was going to enter the armed services, then the Army was the way to go.

In addition to giving me the specialty I wanted, the Army allowed me to submit a "dream sheet" of my three preferred locations for my first assignment.

My first stop after the Army was an 11-week officers' training course — a basic orientation course for officers in the health professions. Although I am told this course is not as intense as the Army basic boot camp, it was very demanding. We were given instruction on Army protocol and regulations and on the expected behavior of officers. We also received rigorous physical training. The physical component of the course cannot be underestimated, because officers must pass annual physical fitness tests and maintain themselves within prescribed weight limits.

Upon completion of my nursing degree, I was commissioned as a second lieutenant in the Army nurse corps, thus starting my military and nursing career ladder, similar to my civilian counterparts. To be commissioned as an Army nurse, I had to meet all eligibility criteria to claim licensure as a registered nurse. However, what is unique about active-duty Army nurses as a group is that we all have BSN degrees. Following the officer basic course, I proceeded on and reported in two weeks to my assigned post at Fitzsimons Army Medical Center in Aurora, Col. At Fitzsimons, I was assigned to a general medical-surgical unit.

I was impressed by the atmosphere in the hospital, especially the mutual respect that was apparent among the staff. I was addressed as Lieutenant Coleman or Ma'am; enlisted men and women were addressed by their rank title, such as Private Johnson. Each person knew his or her job and exactly what was expected. It was apparent that all personnel performed their assigned responsibilities with the knowledge that they were accountable for the outcome. Passing the buck for a mistake was not an option. I liked that. We were judged on our actions and performance.

Despite the military decorum, collegial relationships between physicians and nurses were not inhibited. Almost immediately, I found that physicians and other nurses were friendly and eager for my input as a professional. Doctors routinely discussed my patients with me, asking what I observed, how each patient was reacting to treatments or medications, and what I thought about possible modifications. It was truly a collaborative effort. This attitude even extended to on-call physicians awakened at two or three o'clock in the morning with a question about a patient. Our physicians were always patient, respectful, and concerned, and I was never made to feel that I was annoying a physician or asking a stupid question.

Nurses work eight-hour shifts, five days a week, rotating through nights and weekends. In the Army, shifts always run a little longer than eight hours to ensure that there are no unresolved problems for the next shift. As in any hospital setting, we give reports to the nurses on the next shift, covering the status of each patient and detailing any new treatments or precautions. Any emergencies occurring during the change are the responsibility of the outgoing staff. To cover an unexpected sick call, the supervisor assigns a nurse to stay and cover four hours of the next shift. Also, a nurse from the following shift will be called in four hours early. This can be frustrating, and it can interfere with personal plans. However, the patients need to be taken care of, and this dilemma occurs in civilian nursing as well.

After seven months my orders came through for the specialized OB/GYN practice that I had requested. In the meantime, however, I had rotated through a number of other wards at Fitzsimons, including a women's surgical ward, an OB/GYN unit, a postpartum ward, and a more advanced surgical ward. As a result, I was no longer sure that OB/GYN was my practice choice. So I requested a temporary deferment in entering training and wrote a letter explaining my decision. The Army's ready approval of my delay dispelled another myth that many people have about military service, specifically, that once a person commits to a certain specialty area there is no way out. The Army realizes that people grow and their interests change. The Army also knows that if an officer is unhappy with an assignment, productivity may suffer. So whenever a change of heart occurs, the Army nurse corps tries to accommodate it.

I have since decided that I like the challenge of the operating room. Unlike many civilian hospitals in which training occurs in a more or less on-the-job preceptor model, the Army sends nurses to a school for a formal course. My OR training was an intensive 16-week course at the Brooke Army Medical Center in San Antonio.

On the surgical ward where I currently work, I see a broad range of procedures and conditions: from diaphragm and detached retinal repairs to gallbladder and cataract removals. My responsibilities include day-to-day bedside care, accompanying physicians on rounds, providing preoperative and postoperative education to patients and their families, competing documentation, and performing regular patient assessments. Also, on an evening or night shift, I may be the charge nurse responsible for assigning staff duties. This generally includes other Army nurses and our 91 Bravos who are enlisted soldiers.

Unlike civilian nursing, the Army designates regular periods during the year for specialized training. Some of these are mandatory and some are selective. For instance, I was recently selected to participate in what is known as a C-4 course, or combat care casualty course. This entails eight days of specialized training in battlefield nursing. Field conditions are simulated, so we learn how to assess, triage, and care for severe battlefield trauma and work with limited supplies and resources. Not every nurse is chosen for this type of course.

Initially, the pay of an Army nurse may not be quite equal to that of a civilian nurse, but the difference is more than made up for in benefits. We receive 30 days of paid vacation per year. On-base housing is available and quite comfortable. I live in what could be described as a town-house apartment on base, and subsidies are provided for those who prefer off-base housing. We also receive complete medical and dental care, a monthly food subsidy, cost-of-living increases, and increases for years of service, as well as pay increases for promotion in rank. Continuing education is free, and there are programs that subsidize advance practice studies leading toward a master's degree or a doctorate.

I gave birth to my son Shawn during my second year in the Army, and the medical benefits were comparable to those of any hospital or major corporation. In my second trimester, I was not allowed to work more than 40 hours per week and was given regular breaks on the job. A standard six-week maternity leave can be extended by vacation time, and we are allowed six months following delivery before we are required to pass a physical fitness test or meet weight requirements.

Nurses interested in the military need certain attributes and attitudes. Army life definitely requires a discipline of character and drive to maintain good physical shape. Post assignments change approximately every four years, so the Army nurse must like travel. Communication skills are essential. Not only will I interact with physicians and medical staff, but also with patients who range in rank from private to general. It's important to be able to explain routine care and procedures clearly and in a way that is not overly technical or condescending. Also, the Army places a strong emphasis on achievement; our job performance is reviewed every three months. Finally, the Army expects its nurses to continue to grow professionally during practice. Each nurse is required to earn 20 CEUs yearly from the military in addition to meeting CEU requirements of the state where the nurse practices.

If a nurse enjoys travel, constant challenges, and has a desire to achieve and accept responsibility, the Army should definitely be a consideration. Even if a nurse does not plan a life-long Army career, Army service can provide experience, training, and a degree of responsibility that may not be available as quickly to our civilian counterparts. For me, the Army has been an exceptional choice ... and my career is only beginning.

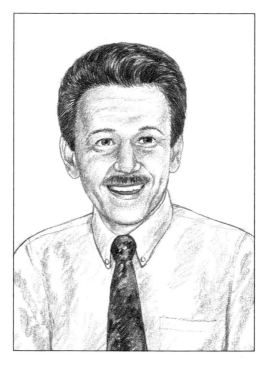

Lieutenant Commander Don Fowler, BSN, RN, is assistant department head of the operating suite at Bethesda Naval Hospital in Maryland.

The Navy Nurse

When I was young, my uncle transfixed me with tales of his life in the Navy — exotic ports and foreign lands. I'm sure his stories had something to do with my decision to shape a career in this service, but what I've found in the Navy goes far beyond the excitement of travel. I've had unparalleled professional opportunities as well as a chance to meet and work with people from every walk of life.

My first experience in the Navy was as an enlisted man. I had enrolled in a one-year laboratory technician program after high school, and when I was unable to find a civilian job immediately, I joined the Navy for four years. Because of my laboratory training, the recruiter was able to guarantee a position in the hospital corps school. This involved an intensive 13-week program that was geared to delivering emergency care in the field: how to stop bleeding, open an airway, start IVs, and relieve pain. In peacetime, corpsmen deliver health care in traditional settings, and so my first health care experiences were in the hospital wards, emergency room, and outpatient clinics.

These four years shaped my career expectations in important ways. As corpsmen, we had to assume an enormous amount of responsibility. In fact, back then we delivered the majority of nursing care with only one registered nurse supervising several units. This staffing pattern is no longer typical, but the challenge was highly motivating for me. It forced me to learn how to make decisions and set priorities effectively. My supervisors respected my judgements and listened to my opinions. This is an aspect of Navy nursing that I believe is unique: If you are willing to go the distance in discharging the responsibilities you are given, the rewards can be enormous. The Navy has unlimited opportunities for people with motivation.

At the end of my first tour of duty, I knew I wanted to become a registered nurse. I had planned to enroll in a Navy program that would send me to school full time, but a temporary cutback of government funds kept me from being able to do this right away. I didn't want to leave the Navy, but my only option was to pursue my education independently. So, instead of reenlisting for another tour of duty, I resigned and used the benefits of the GI bill to enroll in a hospital-based diploma nursing school. At first, I found school frustrating, because few people recognized the knowledge I had gained in four years of experience. Even so, I gained an invaluable academic foundation in the basic sciences.

After graduation, I worked for a year in a general community hospital, an experience that cemented my commitment to the Navy. In that civilian setting, I realized that I enjoy the structure and order of the military. This is not to say that I enjoy rigid, inflexible regulations. But I do believe that military service provides an important exercise in discipline for many people, even if it is only for one tour of duty. The skills and accountability one learns in the Navy can open many career doors in the world of civilian health care.

In 1982, I reenlisted in the Navy as an ensign and a registered nurse, working first on an orthopedic ward and then in a cardiothoracic stepdown unit. This assignment gave me a chance to practice in a highly technical environment with patients who made dramatic changes relatively quickly. After a couple of years, I sought a change and requested assignment as an operating room specialist. This new responsibility called for six months of training and rotation through several different kinds of surgical services. The program is designed to teach nurses how to manage an operating room efficiently, not just to handle the clinical aspects of nursing. This is true because, as of now, Navy nurses do not scrub to work with the surgeons during an operation — OR technicians perform that function. Nurses are far more involved in the overall management of the surgical environment.

After my training was complete, I was given an assignment that is unique to Navy service. I was deployed for several months in the Mediterranean as part of a ship's surgical team. In that capacity, I was responsible for helping maintain an operating room service and clinic for a group of ships, handling routine health complaints or battlefield injuries. Assignments such as this will become available only occasionally, and they add significantly to the variety in a career.

For me, the operating room has been an exciting setting in which to practice nursing. Navy nurses can have substantial influence on their patients, even though they see them only for 10 or 15 minutes before surgery. Even in that brief time, a surprising amount of rapport can be developed — especially in a close-knit military community. For example, it is not uncommon for a nurse to discover that he or she has been stationed at the same facility as a patient and that they have mutual acquaintances. Finding this common ground makes it easy to establish a bond of trust, and it helps alleviate the patient's anxiety.

We serve as the link between the patient and family members, keeping them updated on the progress of the surgery and telling them what to expect afterwards. This relationship is even more important when the patient is a child, because the parents are anxiety-stricken. The contact we have with patients and families is rewarding, but just as important is the fact that each day brings new patients and new challenges; boredom is not a feature of this work.

My career progressed steadily, and I was able to return to college to obtain a BSN. In return for my agreement to serve two additional years on active duty, the Navy footed the bill for two years of full-time study, while continuing to pay my full salary. Without that financial support, I would have found it extremely difficult to study and work full time. My new degree enhanced my credentials as a nurse and led to further promotions.

Now, I work as the assistant department head of the operating suite at the Navy's largest medical facility, in Bethesda. My duties involve more administration than bedside care, but it is far from a dull desk job. I am continually solving problems, from making certain that emergencies are handled properly to seeing that room assignments are coordinated properly. I must make sure that adequate staff, equipment, and anesthesia personnel are available. I communicate with physicians and oversee facility maintenance in terms of supplies and repairs. This requires continuing liaison with the other areas of the hospital. We have 14 operating rooms in all, and the goal with each is to achieve the highest possible efficiency. In a time when health care cost containment is increasingly important, a well-run OR can make a big economic difference.

The Navy recognizes that management skills are an important component of effective leadership. However, high rank and advanced degrees do not automatically confer management expertise. In acknowledgement of this, the Navy nurse corps has begun to use on-the-job training as a way of refining management skills. As part of this program, I belong to a middle managers group that meets once a month so members can share ideas on communication, staff motivation, and related issues.

Nursing today is experiencing considerable change. In the Navy this change is an impetus to develop the full potential of each nurse. The Navy is providing opportunities for its people to accept new responsibilities and new circumstances, while in civilian life most employees must seek change and challenge on their own. And as we all know, it is often easier to settle into a familiar routine. Yet, the Navy relentlessly encourages nurses to look for this challenge. For example, in some surgical cases when local anesthesia is used, our nurses monitor the patient's vital signs, EKGs, and responses to medications. They also administer sedatives intravenously. To help our personnel do their jobs better and to guarantee high-quality care, a group of us developed a reference book that outlines standard protocols for local procedures. In addition, we have access to a PhD nurse who works exclusively in the field of nursing research. Several of his studies have involved OR personnel, and this has given us a chance to get involved in something broader than the delivery of care.

Assignment changes are routine in the Navy, and this helps nurses acquire new skills. The intention is to help you take steps that are just a little above your previous responsibilities. At times, you may feel that you are not ready for the new duty, but I find that I arrive in new assignments with just the right amount of experience. I am confident that my superiors want me to succeed and will help me toward that goal. My work as an assistant department head at Bethesda has led to my new two-year assignment as a department head of the operating suite in Guam. Even though I am going to a smaller facility, this will give me a chance to move up another rung on the ladder.

Because nurses enter the Navy as commissioned officers, they must attend an officer indoctrination course, which covers naval rules and regulations, how officers should conduct themselves, and what responsibilities must be upheld. This course is rigorous, but I am biased in that I think having had enlisted experience first was a plus for me. Just as a corporate executive might have a better understanding of his business if he started at the bottom, naval officers may have a broader perspective if they've had experience as an enlisted person.

In truth, the military aspects of a Navy nursing career seem secondary to me, because my work activities are those of a health care professional. In the OR, we all wear name tags with our ranks, but in taking care of patients and their families, the military persona is secondary. However, when we wear our uniforms outside of work, the military aspect becomes dominant. Even so, the military structure is just that — a structure surrounding a professional job.

A career in Navy nursing can be a life-long career, but that was not always the case. In the beginning, marriage or pregnancy disqualified a nurse for service. Now, of course, families are fully incorporated, and the benefits are very positive. In fact, I met my wife, who also is a registered nurse, in the officer indoctrination school. The Navy makes great efforts to help couples receive assignments to the same duty station. It is not always 100-percent perfect, but there is an awareness of the need to make these accommodations.

The specifics of pay in the military are hard to compare with civilian nursing settings. Civilian nurses have been able to win large financial gains recently because of shortages. But on the outside, my wife and I both would need full-time jobs in order to maintain the lifestyle we enjoy here. As it is now, my wife works part time and is able to spend a great deal of time with our three young children. At this stage of our lives, this seems like a big advantage. In addition to my base pay, I receive housing and food allowances, and all of our medical needs are covered. Beyond those benefits, provisions for military retirement are very attractive.

My experiences in the Navy have been great. I've had the excitement of being on ships and visiting foreign ports, but even more important is the fact that the Navy environment has enabled me to develop personal characteristics that I might not have if left to my own devices. In this stable and predictable community, I've been pushed to turn left occasionally instead of always turning right.

Today, the Navy looks for nurses with baccalaureate degrees and commissions them as ensigns. This new requirement does not restrict the opportunity for advancement, and many nurses are able to study for master's degrees with the Navy's aid. To my mind, this is a clear demonstration of the Navy's eagerness to promote education and career development. Currently, there is increasing interest in nurse specialists, including OR nurses. This is true because as pressure is applied to contain costs, military hospitals are pushing to achieve the higher levels of efficiency that are associated with specialized staff.

My life in the Navy has enabled me to retain enthusiasm for the health care professions. As a result, I wake up each morning eager to go to work. I still find it exciting to realize that my efforts can help patients get better and have an improved quality of life. This is a daily reality in the operating room.

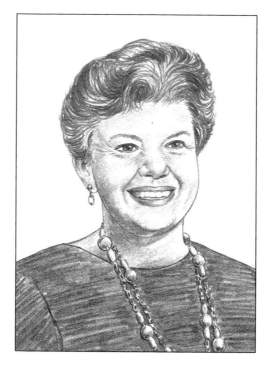

Norma Small, PhD, RN, CRNP,
is coordinator for parish health nursing at
Georgetown University School of Nursing,
and a parish nurse at
Christ Lutheran Church,
in Washington, D.C.

The Parish Nurse

As a nurse and a Christian, I've always been interested in the spiritual dimensions of health care. But until 1986, I'd never heard of parish nursing. Not that it's a new idea — it's just an old one that is being rediscovered.

Because modern medicine places great emphasis on specialization, health care has become a compendium of modular treatments. However, a substantial number of health care professionals are beginning to embrace the concept that health is not simply the absence of disease, but an overall reflection of physical, psychological, social, and spiritual systems. I've found parish nursing fits my ideals of promoting wellness rather than treating sickness.

I had a full nursing career before entering parish nursing. I joined the Army to pay for my last year of school in a Presbyterian hospital diploma program, which I finished in 1957. I worked in general medical nursing, surgical intensive care, and at a burn center. During the Vietnam war I was stationed overseas. While in the Army, I earned my BSN and a master's in medical-surgical nursing.

I had a faculty appointment at the Walter Reed Army Institute of Nursing, where I developed an interest in gerontological practice. After earning a post-master's specialty degree in primary family care, I pursued a PhD in human development with a gerontology focus. In 1981 I joined the Georgetown University School of Nursing faculty to teach in the gerontology master's program.

In 1986, I discovered parish nursing, and three years ago I was given approval to begin a parish health nursing graduate program. The catch was that I had no clinical sites for student experiences. I was reluctant to launch a parish nurse practice at my own church, because I feared it would be difficult for the congregation to separate my nursing role from my already established leadership role. Fortunately, I'd been working with an ecumenical group of churches that addressed problems in my Washington neighborhood. So I walked down the street to the Lutheran church — a 300-member congregation — and was told to go ahead and start a program.

My first hurdle was gaining acceptance for the rather foreign notion of a nurse practicing in a church; people thought they were supposed to go to doctors when they were sick. I worked to reverse this thinking, suggesting instead that my job was to keep them well. But few things move quickly in parish nursing. You plant seeds, water them . . . and then you wait. It took me two years to gain the trust of the congregation.

Health assessment and risk identification are among the major functions I perform. I also offer health education and counseling and train other caregivers. In addition, I serve as liaison with health and community resources. Underlying all these activities is my chief concern — being an effective advocate for vulnerable populations.

Beyond the part I play in caring for individuals or families, I try to help the faith community see itself as part of the health care system, with a responsibility to care for and support its members and the larger community. Parish nurses perform both primary and secondary preventive care, and, although our role is similar to that of a community health nurse, we go further by weaving faith into patient care. When I work with people who face difficult decisions or major life changes, I take a spiritual approach, praying with them for strength and renewal.

When it comes to lifestyle choices, I adhere to the concept that people are the stewards of their own bodies. Estimates say that about 70 percent of premature deaths in the United States stem from lifestyle choices — substance abuse, poor diet, and lack of exercise for examples. And, because 60 percent of Americans say they have a faith that significantly influences their lives, what could be a better way to address the issue of lifestyle changes?

Even if a parish nurse is not a member of the faith community with whom she works, she must understand and commit to its doctrine, integrating beliefs and practices into her nursing. Although I'm Presbyterian, it's easy for me to work in a Lutheran church — the main differences between these denominations are in practice, not belief. When differences are greater, however, ethical conflicts may result. For instance, a nurse in a Catholic church may feel an ethical obligation to tell a woman she has options in pregnancy, but the Catholic church may not be the place to share that information. Or, a nurse may not be able to excuse premarital sex, but still wants to protect the person's health by teaching safe sex. In such cases, the nurse might explain that such behavior conflicts with the church's belief and refer the person somewhere else for help. In each situation, the parish nurse must decide whether spiritual beliefs or nursing concerns take priority. These decisions are highly individual.

Most people need a physical health excuse before they'll come in and ask for help. Adults might want to get their blood pressure checked; a teenager might wander in with a twisted knee from basketball, but then change the subject to a problem at home or at school. Often, people seem more comfortable talking with me than with the pastor about health problems. While the pastor would offer any help he could, he's not specifically trained to make use of community resources. Fortunately I have a good collaborative relationship with the pastor, but it's entirely possible that a parish nurse could run into problems if the pastor felt the nurse was usurping his or her job.

In addition to dealing with individuals, I develop health education programs to address broader topics, including nutrition, AIDS, exercise, caregiving and stress management, making sure they express a holistic approach. Because I'm in touch with various members, I may pinpoint a specific problem that is running through the congregation. For instance, I may present a seminar on arthritis. I've also organized support groups for those who are bereaved or are coping with chronic illness. Recognizing these needs means I must stay in close contact with the members, so I keep office hours and encourage people to drop in. I work the Sunday-morning coffee hour, too, and by noon, I usually have a small entourage following me back to my office.

In general, I serve as a liaison between the congregation and pertinent resources in the community. Instead of reinventing services or resources that already exist, I work with parish committees, health care professionals, and the community to improve resources or make them more accessible to my population. Where there are gaps in service, I may develop a program to address particular problems. For example, I once held an afternoon class for perimenopausal women and their husbands, and it turned into a popular support group. In another instance, I sponsored a meeting between senior high school students and their parents to talk about AIDS. While the teens were reluctant to talk about this directly with their parents, they were comfortable talking in the same room. In fact, I was surprised at how open they were on the subject of sex.

Part of my job is to offer individual and family health counseling — trying to address concerns before they develop into full-blown problems, and helping direct decisions about medications or treatments. However, while I can give people sound health care advice, I must know my limitations and recognize serious conditions that should be referred to a physician, psychotherapist, or the pastor.

Training people to care for themselves and others is one of the parish nurse's most important roles. A community health nurse may train a person to perform a specific activity, but a parish nurse tries to foster a relationship in which the person continues to learn self-care activities. Caring for other people is a central idea in most religions, and because members of a congregation do care about one another, turning to members for caregiving duties is a wise use of human resources.

For the most part, I encourage people to offer simple services — writing a letter or doing the shopping for people who can't do it themselves. Sometimes I've trained volunteers to help care for a home-bound person so the family can take an occasional break. People tend to be afraid of this responsibility, so I teach them such simple skills as helping the patient walk, giving the Eucharist in the home, or communicating with a patient whose sight or hearing is impaired. Most important, I teach the "ministry of presence," which says it is less important to be fully prepared than it is to be fully present.

As part of the caregiving ministry, I'm developing a home care support program. While community home health agencies may be equipped to administer care, they often lack the resources to supervise its delivery. I have trained volunteers to visit patients' homes as an informal way of ensuring quality control. Is abuse taking place, intentionally or unintentionally? Is someone stealing from the patient's home? Is food in the refrigerator spoiled? I'm in an ideal position to intervene with a virtual army of helpers.

I believe my most important function is serving as an advocate for the vulnerable: the young, the old, or those who are disabled in body, mind, or spirit. These people lack the ability or motivation to care for themselves, so it falls to me and the congregation to help.

As parish nursing evolves, we face several concerns. Funding is a major one, because most faith communities and churches are unable to pay the nurse's salary. Consequently, most parish nurses work part time. In many cases, the nurse begins as a volunteer and then is hired when the congregation recognizes her value. Also, some hospitals — especially denominationally affiliated ones — believe that sponsoring a parish nurse is an excellent way to improve their image and to reach out into their communities.

Legal issues are another concern in parish nursing. Currently we're working to define our scope of practice, which varies widely. Some parish nurses consider their role exclusively in the spiritual dimension. Others, especially those who come from acute care settings, feel that if they're not doing something concrete, they're not nursing. Because this interventionist approach may be provided by community health nurses, the trend in parish nursing is toward indirect care. We don't change dressings; we teach how to change dressings. We don't give insulin injections; we teach others how to give them. Our work probably will not expand to encompass the reimbursable tasks that usually are performed by the community health nurse.

In my opinion, parish nursing is not appropriate as a first job. Nurses who enter this field should have a BSN and a background in community health, which usually requires some acute care experience. Postgraduate education is desirable, too, but a parish nurse doesn't necessarily need a master's degree. Even more important than advanced nursing education are good judgement and competence, which come from experience. Because of the autonomy nurses have in this setting, expert assessment and clinical decision-making skills are essential.

And, of course, parish nurses need a strong faith commitment as a theological basis for practice, and they must take a holistic approach to health and to nursing. Parish nurses have tremendous influence on health and healing because they are in a position to redirect a person's focus to the strength of faith. An insulin shot may treat the moment, but we can treat a life.

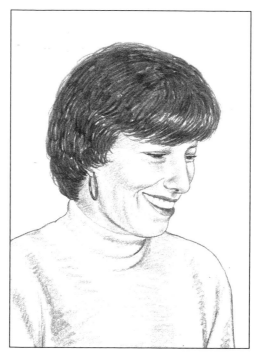

Alice Myerson, MSN, RN,
is a community health nurse and
home infusion therapist.
She works for the Visiting Nurse Service of
New York, in the Bronx.

The Home Care Nurse

Community health nursing, also known as home care nursing, is a highly autonomous and flexible type of practice that regularly challenges a nurse's clinical skills and physical assessment abilities. It is also a practice in which the nurse-patient relationship can become more intimate than in most other nursing environments.

I came to community health nursing after spending 13 years in a hospital environment. I had worked on a general medical-surgical unit, in an emergency room, and spent several years in a medical-surgical ICU. Those experiences helped me acquire a broad base of clinical skills. However, after so many years in the hospital I needed a change, not only in my practice environment, but in the challenges that were available to me. I wanted a clinical practice that would permit me to grow professionally and personally while letting me build upon the extensive clinical skills I had already acquired. Community health nursing seemed perfect.

I made the switch to community health care nursing in 1986, at a time when health care administrators and third-party reimbursers were just beginning to recognize the practical and financial benefits of home care nursing. In many cases, community health nurses can provide home-based care for recovering, chronically ill, and terminal patients that equals the care and services offered in hospitals — and they can do this for significantly less cost. Home care also affords patients a dignity and independence that is impossible in the hospital environment.

The agency I became associated with is the country's oldest and most reputable home care establishment. An experienced nurse can tell a lot about what a work place is like by observing the patients and staff during an introductory tour of the facilities. But because this service operates out of an office complex, I was initially unable to see the interaction between nurses and patients. What did impress me was the way my interview was handled. Instead of telling me what the agency did and explaining how I would fit in, the supervisor asked what I wanted to do. We talked about the type of patients I might like to work with and how I would handle various situations. It was a very relaxed process, more like two colleagues talking with each other rather than a prospective employer measuring an applicant against a set of job criteria. I was also impressed by the camaraderie in the office. Phones were ringing, computers were clicking. But the staff was friendly, smiling and interacting in a purposeful and professional manner.

When I first began, I went through a two-week orientation program that described various protocols, precautions, and standards of practice associated with community health nursing. I also received training in how to practice in the patients' homes. For someone who had practiced so long in the hospital, home care demanded a significant adjustment. Hospitals — especially ICUs — are places of tremendous control. Nurses wear scrubs or white dresses, and our duties are very defined. We control what the patient eats, when he sleeps, when medications are given, when ambulation or exercise occurs. Virtually every component of patients' lives and care are our responsibility. And because we are professionals, we make sure these responsibilities are carried out.

But in the home environment, the nurse is the patient's guest. We wear street clothes and usually can be identified by the rather large blue bags we carry. We do not have the control that is commonplace in the hospital. Nurses in the community have to realize that it is the patient who has autonomy and the final say about treatment and care. Nurses who cannot accept this not only will be frustrated, but they will fail completely. The home environment is a place in which nurses must strike a balance between what they know can be done for the patient and what the patient will accept. Many nurses find this very difficult, but I enjoyed it right away because I believe in the right of individuals to determine their own destinies.

Another important component stressed during my orientation period was communication. At first I thought this was unnecessary for me because I had worked so closely with patients in the past. But I soon discovered that what worked in the hospital — or what I thought worked — did not apply in the home environment. Patient education was one example. In a hospital setting we would sit down with a patient and say something like, "Okay, Mr. Jones, this is your medication. You take four of these three times a day after meals, one of these twice a day before meals, and inject this once every two days or as you feel it is needed." The patient would nod and look as if he followed everything. In fact, he may not have comprehended a word of it, partly because little time is available for education in the hospital and partly because his stress level impeded his ability to learn. In the home environment, what the patient learns is the important thing, not how long it takes to learn it.

In the home we do active teaching. We explain the procedure completely and make sure the patient understands what we will be teaching and why. We show the patient what we want him to do, whether it is following a drug regimen, giving an injection, cleaning a wound, or engaging in rehabilitative activity. Then we have the patient demonstrate what he has learned. In essence, we ask him to teach us so that we can gauge whether he has learned the procedure properly. This process may take one 45-minute visit, or two weeks of daily visits. Each patient is different.

My practice is centered in the South Bronx, New York, a very tough and troubled neighborhood with a reputation for crime and violence. My agency understands this and provides an escort when I go into areas that are dangerous. I am under no pressure to go where I would feel uncomfortable or unsafe. Despite the reputation of the South Bronx, I have never had a real problem. The closest I came was when I pulled up to a curb one afternoon to make a visit. Some young men were on the corner and, without speaking, made it very clear that they didn't want me there. I didn't even think about confrontation. I just left, reported in to my supervisor, and made arrangements to see the patient another time. This situation was atypical in my seven years of community health experience. In general, nurses are highly regarded by the people in the neighborhood because we are seen as positive influences, bringing healing and care to the community. That I speak Spanish helps my relationship with the Hispanic community.

Initially, my practice focused on adult general medical cases. I carried a case load of 20 to 30 patients and made about 36 visits per week. My visits averaged between 45 minutes and two hours. Patients presented with a broad spectrum of conditions and illnesses. I saw patients with diabetes, wounds, and ulcers, elderly people with cardiac and respiratory problems, people requiring dialysis, oncology patients, terminally ill patients, asthmatics, and people who were well except for acute conditions, such as postoperative wound care.

I had seen all these conditions in the hospital, but dealing with them in the home environment presented a completely different challenge. All of a sudden I felt as if I were filling the same role as a country doctor. I had a stethoscope, a blood pressure monitor, a thermometer, and my own five senses. I had to rely on my assessment skills, information provided by the patient's history, and my knowledge of pathophysiology and human dynamics. I have learned to smell urinary tract infections and to listen for what is not said as well as the spoken complaint. This was not a place for someone with limited experience. There was no backup in the field, no one with whom I could discuss my findings. It was just me and the patient.

I was doing more than dealing with the patient's medical presentation: I was caring for the whole patient. I would listen to the person and try to get answers to several questions. How did he feel about his condition, about the role it cast him in with family and friends? Was there support? How safe was the home environment? Were any additional services needed? What could I do to help? Viewing the patient in this perspective and structuring care to address these issues is an important part of home care nursing. Yet, it is difficult, even impractical, to provide this broad care in other settings. In the home, the nurse has the benefit of more time and a more personal level of contact with the patient. The nurse becomes an integral part of the patient's support system. Indeed, the nurse may become the coordinator of that support system. A holistic approach is both appropriate and possible.

Many nurses tend to become too involved in patients' problems, looking for solutions to problems that have no solutions or that could better be resolved by another discipline, such as social work. In the home care environment, it is necessary to know how to triage and enlist other services and how to maintain therapeutic boundaries with the patients. The responsibility of coordinating and facilitating these services can become frustrating because some patients do not have coverage for everything they need and because ancillary services either may not exist or be available. Most, if not all, of my patients receive some sort of public assistance. Medicaid is flexible and will pay for almost anything the patient requires. Medicare is more restrictive and often denies certain services. I never considered insurance policies when I worked in the hospital. Consequently, it is difficult for me to organize my plan of care around what is covered by the insurance policy rather than what is needed by the patient.

Social problems are also part of the home care environment, including alcohol and drug abuse, child abuse, spousal abuse, poverty, violence, hunger, and fear. Much of this can be disturbing to witness. For instance, I had a case where the adult children were physically and emotionally abusing the parents and stealing from them. The father, who was in his late 60s, had organic brain syndrome and was extremely confused. His wife was attempting to care for him, but she was a functional schizophrenic and had problems of her own. The children had left two young grandchildren in her care as well, and both of these youngsters were emotionally disturbed. They lived in a fourth-floor walk-up in a dilapidated building. The apartment's windows were cracked or broken; there was no heat and, sometimes, there wasn't any water. Worst of all, whenever the social security checks arrived, the adult children would take them and cash them, leaving little or nothing for food and other necessities.

I contacted the protective services department right away. At least, I thought, I could get the patient admitted to a nursing home. At best, protective services would stop the thievery and get proper care for all the family members. However, when the adult children discovered I had called, they moved the patient and his family to another borough. As a result, the claim was lost in the protective services system. I had trouble believing people could be so cruel.

I worked in adult care for about three years and then requested a change to our high-tech infusion program. Even though I loved community health nursing, I missed the technological aspects of the

ICU environment. Becoming a home infusion therapist enabled me to get back to more complex treatments and care. I also believed it was time to seek new challenges. I don't believe that any practice can be an end in itself; a nurse must always look for ways to grow professionally.

Our home-infusion program services anyone with an indwelling catheter or a need for home infusions of medications. About 90 percent of our patients are HIV positive, the rest have cancer. A few receive short-term antibiotic therapy for diseases such as osteomyelitis, Lyme disease, or endocarditis. Caring for these patients is very complicated: Their medical therapies are complex, as are their social problems and needs. My goals depend on their needs at any given point in time. Their care demands flexibility because their physical conditions may change rapidly. A person may be independent in his infusion for several months and then suddenly go blind or become more debilitated. Obviously, if this occurs, the plan of care must be revamped, and the nurse must be able to respond to the change.

One of my patients is a four-year-old boy who contracted AIDS because his mother had been infected by her husband. Pediatric infusion patients are a new population for my agency, and I was excited about caring for someone so young. I provide this boy with gamma globulin treatments, which involve a two-hour infusion. Each time I visit I have to insert the catheter, which is difficult because his veins have been stuck so many times they have become very fragile. I monitor him closely during those two hours to keep him from moving too much. We talk and he colors in coloring books. His mother will never become independent in the infusion. My goal is to give the infusion safely at home and keep him out of the hospital as much as possible. His mother is very happy he's being treated at home.

Death is an issue in this area of practice because I lose all of my patients within a few months to a few years. When I was in the ICU, I dealt with death every day, but this feels different. Now, I am much closer to my patients and their families, and it is hard to see them die. At the same time, I try to do all I can to make them comfortable and their last months worthwhile. I know that what I'm doing is meaningful, and that thought keeps me going. My goals for the terminal patients are to relieve pain and provide adequate support to the family to allow the patient to die at home.

Before a nurse enters the field of community health nursing I recommend at least a year of clinical practice in a medical-surgical unit, emergency room, or critical care unit. In this field, assessment skills and the ability to think on your feet mean almost everything. Highly developed communication skills are also essential and the community health nurse must be able to interact with people comfortably, letting them talk ... letting them have control. Naturally, such a nurse must be independent and highly motivated.

Autonomy and flexibility are hallmarks of home care nursing. I am given a specific number of patients to see within a week, but it is up to me to create a schedule and make the visits. I can see them all in two or three days, or I can stretch the visits out over the week. There are no night rotations and few weekends to work. The pay and fringe benefits are excellent. I also get to do a lot of teaching with our staff, especially during the orientation of new nurses. But best of all is the autonomy of my practice and the level of patient contact. At the end of every day, I know I have used my skills and training to touch a life and make a difference.

The Rehabilitation Nurse Educator

Venida Y. Hamilton, MSN, RN, CNA,
is director of nursing education, research,
and systems at the
National Rehabilitation Hospital,
Washington, D.C.

In 1985, when I started my current job as director of nursing education, research, and systems at the National Rehabilitation Hospital in Washington, D.C., the facility was still under construction, and I had to draw on all my experience and creativity to build a nursing education department from the ground up. Not only was the hospital new, it was one of the few on the East Coast that employed nurse educators in the rehabilitation setting. Today, however, rehabilitation education has developed into a career opportunity that offers nurses interesting challenges in many settings.

Nurse educators, particularly those at rehabilitation facilities, must be jacks-of-all-trades. Not only must we plan and implement programs that ensure quality nursing care, but we also need to increase our visibility and demonstrate the value of our work. No hospital or health care facility can compete in today's environment unless its staff members continue to learn. In some facilities, educators are not directly involved in patient care, yet education is an integral component of any rehabilitation program, perhaps even more important than in acute care.

I received a BSN in 1968 and then worked intermittently as a charge nurse in intensive care and medical units until 1972. For the next five years, I worked at a neighborhood health center, providing a combination of outpatient and home health nursing services. There I got my first exposure to nursing education.

As part of my job at the community health center, I was the staff development coordinator, planning and conducting in-service education for professional staff members and paraprofessional personnel. Naturally, those two groups had diverse needs, because the professionals were experienced in health care, while paraprofessionals employed as home health aides might be tackling their first jobs. In-service education for professional staff was built on an established knowledge base and might focus on new equipment techniques or policies and procedures, but the paraprofessionals usually need basic information on specific clinical problems or situations.

While working at the center, I also enrolled in graduate school, following a management track in community health nursing. By the time I finished in 1981, I was employed at the clinical center at the National Institutes of Health as a clinical nurse educator. There, as the educator for the cancer nursing service, I coordinated orientation as well as in-service and continuing education. I organized programs that dealt with chemotherapeutic agents — their administration, side effects, complications, and other cancer treatment modalities. In 1982, I became director of continuing education at the Walter Reed Army Medical Center, and in 1985 I came to the National Rehabilitation Hospital, where I supervise the nurse educators and clinical specialists.

Staff education programs in most health care institutions have three distinct components: orientation, in-service education, and continuing education. Naturally, orientation programs are intended for recently hired nurses. The goal of in-service education is to help nurses keep their skills up to date. Such programs may reinforce existing skills or focus on new techniques. Sometimes they pertain to the hospital's goals in quality assurance or cost containment. They also may be related to a specific nursing problem or based on a staff request.

As either one-time workshops or a series of classes, in-service programs cover topics such as CPR, fire safety, infection control, and documentation. One management series I organized spanned several weeks, during which we reviewed the basic principles of staffing, communication, and leadership. On a more limited scale, we may run a class as many as 20 times to teach our staff how to use a new glucose monitoring device.

Continuing education is meant to impart more advanced knowledge than would be covered in basic nursing education. It is intended to build upon the education and experience of the professional nurse, thereby enhancing practice, education, administration, research, and theory development. This is a broad definition, but continuing education can be very specific, addressing such specific topics as advances in spinal cord injury nursing, cardiac care for the rehabilitation patient, coping with alteration in sexual functioning, and nursing leadership development.

In my current job, I'm responsible for every facet of education, not only of our staff, but of patients as well. I direct the teaching and research activities of my staff, organizing their training and travel, and handling the writing of grant proposals. In addition, each year I usually act as the preceptor for one graduate nursing student in administration or education. My staff conducts a review course for nurses who are preparing to take the examination for certification in rehabilitation. Hospital committee work demands a lot of my time: I serve on committees for quality assurance, continuing education, nursing leadership, research, and strategic planning.

Each year I take my two nurse educators and two clinical specialists on a retreat away from the hospital. We review what we've accomplished in the past year, discuss needed revisions, and devise a plan for the next year's program. With the goals of the nursing service in mind, we determine how we should tailor our educational efforts to help meet its goals. This process involves direct education, but it also must address issues in quality improvement and productivity. We believe that the quality of our education programs has a direct impact on the quality of patient care.

To make sure our education programs are appropriate for our audience, we solicit responses from the nursing staff. We use questionnaires to gather data about programs we've offered in the past and to learn what topics they'd like to see covered in the future. For instance, every three months we ask new nurses what they found most useful in the orientation program and how they've applied what they learned.

We used to have a two-week orientation program. The first week introduced nurses to the facility, the second covered clinical concepts in rehabilitation nursing. This course is specific to our institution and goes beyond the basic nursing curricula. However, after talking to attendees we discovered that most nurses wanted to start work on the unit sooner than we were letting them. Many felt the course would have more value if it were given after a month or so on the job. Based on this feedback, we retooled the program so that new nurses now get four days of straight orientation, then begin working on the unit. After they have gained a month of experience, they take the rehabilitation course.

Our course offerings also have been influenced by the realities of cost containment. For example, our rehabilitation patients are now admitted with more acute problems than ever before. In response to this, we sponsored a program on acute care management of the rehabilitation patient, and it turned out to be our most popular course. We're also seeing more patients with cardiac problems, so we recently conducted a workshop called "The Hurting, Healing, Loving Heart."

Since we've begun to automate our service through computerized information systems, my department has been involved in training nurses to use the new equipment. For instance, we now use computers to handle admissions and discharges, bed assignments, and clinical data records. This makes the information easier to record and track.

Each year, nurses must review their knowledge and skills in CPR, infection control, fire safety, and, for RNs, mock code blues. However, when we scheduled these in-service seminars separately throughout the year, we had an inadequate response rate — roughly 40 percent. To counter that, we began to offer all the topics during a single review day. Attendance is mandatory and has been nearly perfect.

My staff does quite a bit of one-on-one education, and in those instances I serve as a resource. For instance, a nurse might ask one of my staff for information on how to work with a certain population of patients. In turn, the staff member might ask me to suggest a good background resource. Some subjects lend themselves to games, and we have modified *Monopoly*® and *Jeopardy* to suit our educational needs. In fact, one of my staff has published an article on the use of board games in teaching.

When it comes to making clinical choices in educational programs for master's-level nurses, my staff clears things through me and keeps me informed, but they don't require hand holding. However, when we sit down to discuss program development and planning, no decisions are unilateral. Instead, we brainstorm and reach a consensus.

In my role as an administrator, I do very little direct teaching within the hospital. However, I do make presentations at state and national meetings. For instance, I've presented programs on training rehabilitation technicians, keeping a staff development service viable, managing grants, and precepting students.

I've become an informal career counselor for the nursing staff. When nurses want to go back to school — either for their BSNs or master's degrees — they often talk with me first. Last year, two of our nurses returned for their baccalaureate degrees and arranged to complete their leadership practicums under my supervision. I enjoy that, because it gives me a chance to show staff nurses "the big picture" of the management role. Occasionally, I allow staff members to follow my activities informally, just to let them gain some insight into a supervisor's position. For nurses who are having a hard time understanding why certain decisions are made, this can prove very helpful.

Occasionally, I find myself involved in helping my staff members realign their priorities and focus their energies appropriately. It's easy for a clinical specialist to get overburdened with work on hospital committees. This is especially true of rehabilitation specialists, because they have such an interdisciplinary focus. They're bombarded with requests, and we collaborate on setting priorities. This process often boils down to the answer to a single question: Is there a clinical or political benefit to serving on a certain committee? If the answer is no, we're better off directing our energies elsewhere.

Because rehabilitation nursing depends so heavily on an interdisciplinary approach, I've tried to make our programs reflect that. In acute care, the nurse and the physician are the principal caregivers. In rehabilitation, however, the nurse, physician, physical therapist, occupational therapist, and other clinicians form a team. This team concept is new and sometimes intimidating to nurses who have not practiced in a rehabilitation setting. To assist our nurses in assimilating this concept, our orientation process incorporates classes that describe the nurse's role on an interdisciplinary team. And, using the role-play technique, we have coordinated in-services on assertiveness and stress management.

This job requires a person who can communicate effectively with professionals at various levels, inside and outside of the institution. To be effective in my work, for example, I must be able to negotiate successfully and to market my staff's services. A director of nursing education must be master's prepared, certified in nursing education, and preferably, certified in nursing administration.

Educators often find themselves in the position of justifying the value of what they do, and if an institution wants to downsize, the nurse educator position may be one of the first to be cut. Fortunately, the work we do in this department is appreciated. In our hospital newsletter, *Roses,* staff members can pat others on the back for a job well done. Last year a nurse applauded the nursing education department. She thanked us for the wonderful classes she'd been attending. She believed we had made a difference in her life, and I think that is the ultimate reward for any teacher.

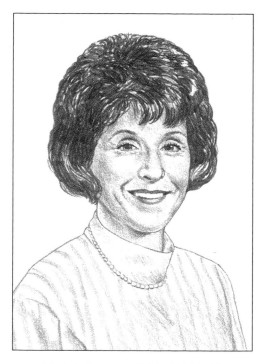

Virginia K. Saba, EdD, RN, FAAN,
is an associate professor at the
Georgetown University School of Nursing in
Washington, D.C.

Informatics: An Overview

Informatics is derived from the French word *informatique,* and it refers to all aspects of the computer milieu. It is a new specialty that encompasses all the health sciences and professions. Nursing informatics is particularly concerned with the application of information and computer technology to enhance the use of knowledge in our profession.

Nursing informatics has emerged as a new nursing specialty concerned with standardizing documentation, improving communication, supporting the decision-making process, developing and disseminating new knowledge, enhancing the quality and effectiveness with which health care is delivered, empowering clients to make health care choices, and advancing the science of nursing.

In 1991, the American Nurses Association designated nursing informatics as a practice specialty and defined it as one that ". . . integrates nursing science, computer science, and information science in identifying, collecting, processing, and managing data to support nursing practice, administration, education, and research; and to expand nursing knowledge. The purpose of nursing informatics is to analyze information requirements; design, implement, and evaluate information systems and data structures that support nursing; and identify and apply computer technologies for nursing."

The demand for expertise in nursing informatics is strong and growing. This is evidenced by the variety of organizations that are developing guidelines specifying what information is needed for clinical communication, documenting the nursing process, managing decision making, accreditation, and reimbursement, and for demonstrating the quality of patient care.

As early as the 1950s, nursing informatics emerged with the introduction of computers in nursing. As the data-processing industry expanded, so did the use of computers in the health care industry. The early uses of computers in hospitals and other health care agencies were for business functions. However, by the mid-1960s, computers were being used for selected applications in patient care. In the 1970s, the introduction of on-line terminals, data communication, and real-time processing made it possible to employ computers in integrated hospital-wide information systems. Such systems included nursing applications, several of which were the forerunners of nursing information systems that exist today.

With the introduction of the personal computer in the 1980s, computing power became available to individual nurses. Moreover, user-friendly generic software allowed nurses to develop their own application programs, thereby reducing their dependence on professional programmers. Furthermore, microcomputers could be linked to each other in networks, as well as to existing hospital computer systems.

The 1990s brought computers to the patient's bedside and to all settings where nurses practice. Today, they are viewed as technological tools that make it possible to process increasing amounts of complex patient data and to improve the quality of care. Clinical workstations, computerized record keeping, and high-speed communications are increasing the demand for nursing informatics specialists.

Informatics specialists are involved in all phases of nursing information systems — from design, development, and implementation to training, maintenance, and evaluation. Their systems are used to administer nursing services, manage the delivery of patient care, and support nursing education and research.

In administering nursing services, informatics specialists use patient classifications in developing programs for staffing, scheduling, personnel management, risk management, and quality assurance. In managing patient care, they develop programs for care planning, order entry, results reporting, vital signs and symptoms documentation, and an array of other specific applications.

As support for nursing education, computer-based materials are being developed to teach students as well as staff and faculty. These include computer-assisted instruction and interactive video materials. However, microcomputer software packages are also being used to assist in the teaching process itself through word processing (for papers), spreadsheets (for budgets), database management (for research), and graphics packages (for illustrations).

In the support of nursing research, informatics specialists are involved in research in designing and developing information systems that address nursing phenomena, decision support, and cost and delivery of nursing care. They use computer systems for searching the literature, processing data, analyzing statistics, and disseminating research findings.

A nursing informatics specialist can be helpful wherever nurses practice and in educational settings wherever nursing students are being taught and research is being conducted. The largest number of these specialists work in hospitals, where they also are known as systems nurses, systems coordinators, nurse analysts, and an array of other titles. They usually are employed by the department of nursing at the level of supervisor or coordinator. Others, including nurse analysts, are employed by the computer department, where they interface with patient care units and are involved in the life cycle of the system. The number of specialists in any hospital depends on the size of the hospital and the scope of the computer systems involved.

Information systems specialists have numerous duties, chief of which is to represent the department of nursing in implementing a hospital information system. Their activities include serving as liaison among the nursing and computer departments and all other departments that are involved in implementing or maintaining the hospital information system; educating, orienting, updating, and training nurses and other unit personnel to use the system; providing support to nurses and other personnel using the system; and representing nursing on committees involved in the development and implementation of nursing information systems.

The major liaison activities of these specialists involve troubleshooting on all patient care units where the computer system is installed to ensure that it performs as planned. The specialists also assist in modifying the format of terminal screens to make them nurse friendly. They consult with system users and developers and review file structures.

Teaching staff to use the system is another responsibility of these specialists, and it includes lectures, demonstrations, orientation through hands-on training and reference manuals (which they have prepared) to provide backup for applications.

Clinical support is provided through the assistance of staff nurses and other users on patient units where the system has been installed. The specialists respond to users' questions, a process of trial and error that goes on continuously. They support the applications being developed and tested, they are involved in developing new nursing applications, they help make the systems easier to use, and they have responsibility for research, evaluation, and maintenance.

The last major activity of these specialists includes serving on hospital committees responsible for the life cycle of a system — from design and development to implementation and maintenance. They provide feedback to the nursing department and represent the demands of nursing with others who are involved in each system.

There are no educational requirements for the nurse interested in nursing informatics. However, hospitals that employ such specialists generally require a bachelor of science degree in nursing, formal courses in computer technology, and experience in a clinical nursing specialty. Computer literacy is a given, as is knowledge of computer hardware, software, database management, and data processing, including the ability to use microcomputer software. Both verbal and written communication skills are requisite, and so are interpersonal skills.

Because of the recommendation by the National League for Nursing that computer technology be integrated into the curriculum, most schools of nursing offer some computer courses. Indeed, several schools of nursing now offer nursing informatics specialty education at the baccalaureate, master's, and doctoral levels. At least four academic programs prepare registered nurses in nursing informatics at the graduate level: three of these grant a master's of science degree, and one program awards a doctor of philosophy degree. Other graduate programs are being planned at academic centers nationwide. In addition, nondegree educational programs are available. Examples are, the Summer Informatics Institute at the University of Maryland, a postdoctoral fellowship program at the University of Utah, and the nurse scholars programs offered by HBO and Company in Atlanta, Ga. Also, several conferences and workshops are offered annually by a wide range of sponsors.

In 1986, the American Nurses Association (ANA) initiated the Council on Computer Applications in Nursing (CCAN). The council and the newly formed ANA Steering Committees on Databases to Support Nursing Practice are involved in formulating national policies on nursing informatics. Together they work with federal agencies and other organizations concerned with issues that have an impact on nursing systems.

In 1987, the National League for Nursing (NLN) also initiated a Council for Nursing Informatics, which has responsibility for establishing criteria for integrating nursing informatics in nursing education curricula. The American Medical Informatics Association (AMIA) has a working group (formerly known as PS-G) that focuses on interpreting nursing informatics for the medical profession. Still another organization is Working Group 8, which functions within the International Medical Informatics Association (IMIA). Working Group 8 has been in existence for over 10 years and has set international guidelines for nursing informatics practice and education.

Specialty forums and materials: Several annual conferences provide a forum for nursing informatics specialists to present papers, demonstrate applications, and describe research and advances in the field. The major ones include the annual Symposium on Computer Applications in Medical Care, the annual Rutgers Nursing Informatics Conference, the ANA Biannual Conference Software and Demonstration Theater, the NLN Biannual Computers and Nursing Research Informatics Conference, and an annual New York University Medical Center seminar.

CCAN has published several monographs and has one in press that outline the criteria and content for the four major aspects of nursing informatics — clinical practice, education, research, and administration:

- *Computer Design Criteria for Systems that Support the Nursing Process* (1988)
- *Computers in Nursing Education* (1987)
- *Computers in Nursing Research: A Theoretical Perspective* (1991)
- *Next-Generation in Nursing Informatics Systems* (1993)
- *Computers in Nursing Administration* (1994)

The NLN Council for Nursing Informatics also has published documents that focus on the educational criteria for introducing nursing informatics into nursing curricula. These documents form the basis of nursing informatics.

Computers in Nursing is a refereed journal that focuses on nursing informatics. The ANA Council Newsletter and *Nurse Educator's Microworld* provide additional periodic information. The following textbooks offer comprehensive information about nursing informatics:

- Ball MJ, Hannah KJ. *Using Computers in Nursing.* Norwalk, Conn.: Appleton, Century-Crofts; 1984.
- Ball MJ, Hannah KJ, Jelger UG, Peterson H, eds. *Nursing Informatics: Where Caring and Technology Meet.* New York: Springer-Verlag; 1988.
- Hannah KJ, Guillemin EJ, Conklin DN, eds. *Nursing Uses of Computers and Information Science.* New York: Springer Publishing Company; 1985.
- Saba VK, McCormick KA. *Essentials of Computers for Nurses.* Philadelphia: JB Lippincott; 1986.
- Saba VK, Rieder K, Pocklington D, eds. *Nursing and Computers: An Anthology.* New York: Springer-Verlag; 1989.
- Werley HH, Grier MR, eds. *Nursing Information Systems.* New York: Springer Publishing Company; 1981.

As of 1991, there were approximately 5,000 registered nurses who have identified nursing informatics as their area of interest. This contrasts with 1981, when 15 nurses met as a group during the annual symposium of computer applications in medical care. Representation at the 1991 symposium was as follows: ANA, 206; AMIA, PS-G Group, 120; Capital Area Roundtables on Informatics in Nursing, 400; Council on Nursing Informatics, 389; *Computers in Nursing* subscribers, 3,895.

The ANA's Council on Computer Applications in Nursing has established a subcommittee to develop the scope of practice, guidelines, and standards in order to offer certification of a new nursing specialist called a *nurse informatician.* Their work is scheduled for completion by 1995.

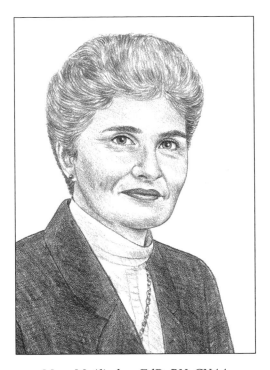

Mary McAlindon, EdD, RN, CNAA,
is assistant to the vice president
for nursing informatics at
McLaren Regional Medical Center,
Flint, Michigan.

The Nurse and Informatics

Nursing informatics involves the triad of data, information, and knowledge as it relates to nursing applications. Informaticians collect and process data into patterns of information, and then apply those patterns in four major areas: clinical practice, education, research, and administration. Nurse informaticians develop systems that help other nurses administer services, manage patient care, and support nursing education and research. The field integrates a nursing science background with the information science procedures of data collection and processing, and uses computer science as its tool. While this still is a developing field, opportunities are growing quickly as technological advances in clinical workstations, computer-based patient records, and high-speed communication systems demand more and more nurse informaticians.

It was 1980, personal computers were just coming on the scene, and the hospital I worked for had just purchased one. We were on technology's cutting edge. The trouble was that nobody knew how to use a personal computer.

I'd just finished a master's degree in education at the University of Michigan and had taken a position as the assistant director of nursing for quality assurance at McLaren Regional Medical Center. Because my job required that I use this computer, I called the university and found someone to help me and my staff understand programming and statistics, data gathering, and data entry. Thus began my infatuation with nursing informatics.

The terms *nurse informatician* and *computer nurse* are often used interchangeably, but to be accurate, a computer is only the tool a nurse informatician uses. The real focus of the job is collecting and collating data into patterns and then interpreting those patterns to produce knowledge that can be applied. But with vast amounts of health care data (that double every two years), the computer has become a necessary medium.

One of my first projects was to organize a patient-classification system, categorizing patients according to the acuteness of their conditions and using that information to determine staffing needs. Now, this system has been refined, expanded, and blended into a scheduling program that tells us how many nurses are needed on each unit for the shift.

While we learned to use the computer, these functions were performed manually. But the computer enabled us to track much more information. We could calculate nurse productivity, and we could follow trends in our patient population. Because I was in quality assurance, I also found it useful to pinpoint when, under what circumstances, and with whom medication errors occurred. Armed with such unprecedented particulars, we were able to troubleshoot the problem at the source.

In one project, we tracked the incidence of patients falling out of bed, recording the sex and age of the person who had fallen. We found that a significant number of these unfortunate patients were elderly women who were getting up to go to the bathroom at night—every three hours—and we put stickers on their wheelchairs and charts identifying them as potential "fallers."

Another study investigated the hospital's use of tympanic thermometers, which had been purchased for $400 each. The physicians were complaining that these instruments gave inconsistent readings so we sought to determine whether they were indeed unreliable. First we ran tests on healthy people, using both tympanic and oral thermometers and comparing the results. Then we turned to patients. Because a tympanic thermometer registers core temperature, it should read one degree higher than a conventional thermometer. However, in one unit the readings were lower. As a result, we concluded that technique was at least part of the problem. After we taught users how to seat the thermometer in the ear, the physicians' complaints stopped — and our expensive thermometers stopped going to waste.

Another aspect of my job in informatics is handling computer tasks for the nursing department. I'm in charge of installing new equipment and training the nurses to use it. Also, I test new software to see if it will work for our applications. In addition, I help design clinical information systems, selecting and gathering data, building databases, and teaching people to use them.

In one such system, laboratory workers enter test results into a computer, and the information is immediately available via terminals at each nursing station. We're planning to install similar databases for pharmacy and radiology. This will enable other departments (eg, nutritional services and physical therapy) to access information that can help them do their jobs better and more efficiently. As an added benefit, the data we amass becomes a resource when we're conducting studies. Nurses also use computers to enter and look up admission, discharge, and transfer information.

Nursing informatics is subdivided into various applications, including education, administration, clinical practice, and research. For instance, I collect data on how much we paid for sick leave and how many nurses were needed to care for patients on each unit. These raw data are synthesized into statistics that are helpful to hospital administrators. In addition, I keep monthly summaries of absenteeism, medication errors, and productivity in nursing units.

Documenting nursing practice is the next challenge for nursing informatics. Pharmacists dispense thousands of drugs in variable dosages and frequencies for many illnesses. That's a large task, but a rather well-defined one. It is somewhat more difficult to define activities that take place in nursing. We give medications and change dressings, and that's easy enough to document. But we also monitor patients — that's where it gets tricky, because details of this activity don't necessarily get charted. Currently, nurses on the national scene are working to give us a lexicon and taxonomy for our work. Someday, this may make it possible to standardize our work and, thus, capture its minutiae in usable documentation. One possible solution is establishing "clinical pathways" that set guidelines for the progress of care. In other words, nurses would set goals for patients and document whether those goals are achieved.

How this documentation is accomplished is another question. Bedside terminals have been proposed, but I think a better alternative is hand-held computers that would automatically download into the main computer. For one thing, 10 hand-held units cost less than 40 bedside terminals. Besides, not all care is delivered at the bedside.

Technology will revolutionize nursing informatics. Eventually, I suspect we'll see a nationwide record of patients. This database will contain a person's entire medical record and will help ensure continuity of care. People also may carry their medical records with them — on plastic cards in their wallets. As informatics catches on, we'll surely conduct interhospital studies that will enlarge the data pool. Of course, the costs of technology may slow this progress: I'm still working to furnish nurses with modems they can use to access online databases and the latest patient care information.

For people interested in nursing informatics, it's crucial to have a strong nursing background, which will be invaluable when it comes to synthesizing clinical information. During this period, try to serve on hospital committees that gather and use data to make decisions. Take classes to become comfortable with computers. Even at this stage, begin making critical evaluations, considering how more information could make things work better.

After building a strong clinical foundation, seek employment working with information systems, translating data into specific nursing applications. In large hospitals, it's possible to serve as a liaison between nursing and the information systems department — listening to nursing's clinical needs and working to install data-processing systems.

The top people in nursing informatics are systems analysts, the creative thinkers who can design computer systems. These professionals have vision that goes beyond popular thinking, and their activities extend beyond the walls of any one hospital. At this level, informaticians practice in their own specialty and are concerned about how their work relates to the nursing profession at large.

I recently finished work on a doctoral degree in education, and for my dissertation in instructional technology, I prepared an interactive video — an educational application that was tailor-made for nurses in the clinical setting. Outside the educational and hospital arenas, informaticians might work in public health departments, accrediting agencies, professional organizations, or even for hardware and software vendors who need nurses to sell and provide design input. Consulting is another option for nurses who have had the experience of installing information systems.

I spend much of my time with staff nurses who are aware of problems that may be occurring or who can suggest bits and pieces or categories of data that I should be following. They let me know if systems are breaking down. For instance, if the anesthesiologist is complaining that he isn't getting lab results of preadmission testing soon enough, I'll probably hear about it from a staff nurse.

It's important for nurse informaticians to be intelligent, inquisitive, diplomatic people who are eager to learn. They should not be intimidated by technology, yet they should be able to balance the application of technology with human needs. In this field, it's not necessary to be a mathematical genius, but it is necessary to be a thinker. In fact, all nurses spend time recording and accessing data. The problem is that they're not getting to the information level of the data-information-knowledge pyramid. Instead, the data are in bits and pieces, and nurses do not have an opportunity to see the parts as a whole and to understand how they might bear on patient care. This will change. And once it does, nurse informaticians may change the entire character of nursing.

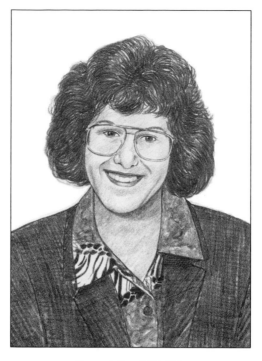

Sara Adler, MS, RN,
is patient care manager at
Beth Israel Hospital,
New York, New York.

The Case Manager

In the past, the career path open to bedside nurses led to administration or academia. Both provided opportunities and new challenges, but they drew experienced nurses away from patient care. Many wondered if this was the best use of their skills and knowledge. And what about the hospital-based bedside nurse who wanted to move up the career ladder but didn't want to pursue management, teaching, or research activities?

Case management is an alternative nursing role that resolves questions like these. This system of delivering care shifts the nurse's responsibilities from bedside primary care to indirect participation in patient care. It differs significantly from function-oriented nursing by allowing experienced nurses to act as coordinators, monitoring continuity of care and managing the scheduling and implementation of ancillary tasks and services. Effective case management can reduce the duration of a patient's stay in the hospital and cut costs without diminishing the quality of care. As a career option, case management bypasses traditional administration and academics but offers new practice challenges that are not too far removed from the bedside.

The case manager's role is to free staff nurses from duties that take time away from hands-on, bedside care. We schedule appointments for lab tests, imaging studies, and physical and occupational therapy, and then we perform any necessary follow-up. We make rounds and consult with physicians, and we routinely evaluate the status of patients. When a patient's stay is drawing to a close, we work with discharge planners to make sure there is adequate access to continued care. Providing education and counseling for patients and their families is also our province. The best way to explain this system is to show how it works in practice.

I am the patient care manager for an orthopedics unit. Almost all patients in the unit are elderly, and about 65 percent rely on Medicaid or Medicare. My average case load is between 15 and 20 patients, and I select my own patients. In general, I choose patients who have the most difficult and, thus, the most time-consuming presentations. Many have broken hips, legs, or clavicles. Most of these cases are complicated by other diseases that may have nothing to do with orthopedics (eg, heart disease).

The circumstances that led to these complex presentations vary. Some patients may have come to the hospital with one ailment and then sustained a fracture as a result of a fall. Others were transferred

301

from a nursing home for treatment of a broken bone. The majority of our patients have been living with chronic diseases — ulcers, diabetes, arthritis, or pulmonary problems — often without adequate health care. They may have been unwilling or financially unable to seek treatment for their conditions. Thus, the severe fall that finally brought them to the hospital is often a signal of general deterioration. These patients need help with a great deal more than their fractures.

Every day, I review the charts of new admissions. My four years of experience as a staff orthopedic nurse helps me identify patients with complex needs. But to refine the process, we have also created over 70 multidisciplinary action plans (MAPs) that provide a very clear indication of the range and depth of care a patient requires.

MAPs are diagnosis-specific algorithms — sample treatment plans that detail the patient's expected daily care and outcomes. MAPs encompass more than traditional nursing considerations because they were created in collaboration with several departments, including medicine, nursing, social work, allied health, pharmacy, rehabilitation services, and discharge planning. Although it is meant only to be a guideline, a MAP gives the case manager an indication of which services a patient will need. In reality, the plan of care for every patient must be modified to reflect actual treatment outcomes.

From the moment I take a case, I begin planning for the patient's discharge. The medical facts alone provide a reasonable assessment of the patient's postdischarge abilities. But soon after taking a case I meet with the patient's social worker to share this information and to learn about the environment the patient lived in before entering the hospital. This is important, because it may have a bearing on the recommendations I make for care after discharge. For instance, if extensive rehabilitation is necessary and the patient lives alone, I will probably schedule a visiting nurse, arrange for live-in help, or make arrangements for the patient to enter a nursing home. If I can anticipate these circumstances, I can involve rehabilitation physicians and physical and occupational therapists from the very first day of admission. These professionals meet the patient, explain a little of what we will be trying to achieve postoperatively, and begin creating their own rehabilitation plans. Thus, the patient is on their schedule, so there won't be any delays in beginning therapy after discharge.

Throughout the patient's stay I serve as the link between the patient's family and the health care team. I meet with the family and explain the patient's problem and the care he or she will receive. Then I describe the progress we expect and what is likely to happen after discharge. This is particularly important if the physician is unable to meet with the family on the day of admission. I offer my business card and tell the family to call me with any other questions or concerns. This eliminates many of the frustrations that are common when people are simply trying to find out what is happening with their loved one. They can turn to me — the case manager — and get straight answers without delay.

In the postoperative phase, I carefully monitor and assess the progress of my patients. I make rounds each day with the physician and care team, consult with rehabilitation professionals, and record my observations in the patient's chart. I want to be sure patients are receiving the care they need on schedule. I also want to verify that no unnecessary tests and resources are being used.

After their discharge, I follow patients to see that the resources I arranged are in place and working well. This continuing follow-up enables us to solicit feedback on the success of our own efforts. Was the education we provided in the hospital retained? Is there anything else we could do during the inpatient period that will improve patients' discharge experience?

From a nursing and medical perspective, we have found that multi-disciplinary patient care improves the continuity of patient care. Because of the trend toward flex-time, it has become less likely that one nurse will maintain contact with the same patient throughout the hospital stay. However, the patient care manager is on the job Monday through Friday. She is a steady presence, not only for the patient, but also for staff nurses and other health care professionals who are working with the patient.

After this system had been in place for several months, we asked the staff nurses if they would prefer carrying eight or nine patients with a case manager, or revert to the old system, carrying fewer patients but also assuming case-management responsibilities. Overwhelmingly, they voted for the separate case manager system. Why? Because the system freed them from paperwork and follow-up duties and made it possible for them to concentrate on what they knew was most important: direct bedside care.

Hospital administrators favor the system because it has contributed to reductions in hospital stay and overall costs while maintaining or even increasing the quality of patient care. In fact, before we instituted case management in orthopedics, patients were hospitalized an average of 9.8 days. Now, due to case management and other improvements in patient care, our average length of stay has dropped to 5.5 days.

From a career standpoint, case management has been great for me. Before my current assignment, I had taken an administrative position. The job offered plenty of new challenges, but I really missed having patient contact. Today, I have the best of both worlds. I have been able to stay clinically involved while moving along in my career with new responsibilities. And the new skills I'm learning — assertiveness, communication, and negotiating — will be invaluable as I move up the career ladder.

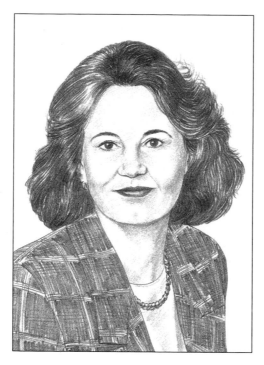

Lillie Shortridge, EdD, RN, FNP, FAAN, is professor and director of the Center for Nursing Research and Clinical Practice at Pace University, Pleasantville, New York, and visiting professor of international nursing at Columbia University School of Nursing, New York, New York. She also is visiting professor of nursing science at the University of Utrecht, The Netherlands.

Managing a Health Center

The boundaries between nursing and medicine shift dramatically depending on the setting. For instance, when I was studying for my baccalaureate degree at Berea College in Kentucky, I gained some experience in the Frontier Nursing Service, a program that used nurses to deliver primary care in rural areas. So when I joined Columbia Presbyterian Medical Center after graduating in 1968, I was surprised to discover that many functions I had learned and was competent in performing were considered part of the medical domain, strictly off limits to nurses. I quickly discovered how arbitrary the doctor-nurse boundaries are, and while I think it's important to have a healthy respect for those boundaries in one's workplace, it's also important to realize that they do not have to wall nurses off from independence in patient care.

It was that belief that sparked my interest in nurse-managed health centers such as the one I run at Pace University. I reasoned that such an environment would allow nurses to broaden their practices, while providing desperately needed access to primary care.

At Columbia, I began teaching at the school of nursing while working toward my MEd in adult medical-surgical nursing. Afterwards, I worked toward an EdD in adult health and education, which I completed in 1977. During these years, I also worked in the hospital's medical-surgical unit, first as a staff nurse and then as head nurse. This hospital experience was important to me, because I believe teachers in the classroom should be able to refer to their first-hand experiences, not just textbooks.

After earning my doctorate, I completed a postdoctoral fellowship at the University of Colorado, working mainly in family primary care. I was motivated by the concept that true comprehensive care involves the family as well as the patient. I wanted to be prepared to care for any member of a family and feel knowledgeable about family dynamics. After this year-long program, I accepted a teaching position at the University of California, San Francisco, where I developed and implemented a family nurse practitioner program.

In 1981, I decided to move back to the East Coast and found a position with a nurse-managed clinic at the Pleasantville campus of Pace University. Originally, the clinic was meant to be a teaching site where nurse practitioner students could develop their skills, and where faculty members could maintain their clinical practices. However, it was clear that the demand for the clinic's services was increasing and that its health care function in the community was just as significant as its academic mandate.

Thus, when I came to Pace I wanted to expand this small clinic into a viable health care system. To accomplish that, I helped develop the Center for Nursing Research and Clinical Practice and secured grants to study and implement the transition from a small practice unit run by the Lienhard School of Nursing to a year-round system that would become the university's health care service, treating students, faculty, and staff. It took six years, but by the end of the grant in 1990 we'd established nurse-managed clinics on all Pace campuses. With funding from other grants, we also developed two outreach programs involving nurse-managed clinics: one for the homeless in Yonkers, N.Y., and one for the elderly in New Jersey.

For the most part, nurse-managed clinics are run by a core staff of master's-prepared nurse practitioners. Some also employ RNs or LPNs. At Pace, we have physicians on retainer, and we pay them as consultants. While it's true they're at the other end of the telephone, they're not at our side. Thus, the nurse assumes most of the responsibility for assessment and decision making. And, unlike nurse practitioners who work in conjunction with a physician, at a nurse-managed clinic the nurses are in charge of hiring and firing physicians — a fairly significant twist of the traditional power structure.

To some degree, my responsibilities and privileges overlap those of a physician: I can order lab tests and write a prescription if warranted. The greatest difference between my role and that of a physician is the amount of time spent with the patient and the emphasis on health promotion. In truth, I've found that most patients don't differentiate between a physician and a nurse practitioner. To them, a provider of care is a provider of care. However, a doctor's office and a nurse-managed clinic are very different settings when it comes to delivering care.

At our university clinic, for example, the focus is on preventive care, and we have established programs to promote those objectives. We give group lectures on such topics as exercise or diabetic care. We also offer personal health management programs in which we work with individual patients in the areas of physical fitness, nutrition, and stress management. We set goals with the patient, meet six times over a period of several months, and then evaluate the success of the program. Many patients enroll in all three programs. That kind of comprehensive care simply isn't available in a traditional doctor's office.

Obviously, the emphasis must be different in our clinic for the homeless. It makes little sense to teach nutrition principles when the person you're teaching can't buy food, or to encourage exercise when the person is deprived of sleep. Instead, at the shelter we encourage interaction with patients in the hope that it may help resolve some of their socioeconomic problems. During the course of a routine history and physical, for example, I may notice an old injury. By asking about it, I may get the person talking about his prison record, crises in his life, problems he's facing now. Armed with this information, I might be able to help the patient begin thinking about ways to break the cycle of hopelessness in his life.

In providing health care to the homeless, we must anticipate the obstacles raised by their circumstances. A homeless person being treated for tuberculosis is likely to need help with figuring out where to keep his supply of drugs, how to pay for them, and how to remember when to take them. The lack of security and continuity in the lives of homeless people make it difficult to maintain the semblance of a routine.

The traditional 15-minute office visit often does not allow sufficient time for comprehensive care. As a result, we don't schedule appointments so close together. I may have to spend 15 minutes with one patient and an hour with the next. We emphasize health care that combines health screening, patient education, and counseling with any treatment. And if we must refer a patient to a physician, we stay involved. We send the patient to the doctor with a list of questions, and we continue our education and counseling. We offer support to the family, and we ensure continuity of care by remaining in touch with the physician and the hospital nurses.

Because of my certification as a family therapist and a family nurse practitioner, I am interested in the effect family dynamics may have on the patient's health. So when taking a history and performing a physical examination, I take the time to learn something about my patient as a person. For example, chronic headaches may be related to marital or parenting problems. When I suspect that the physical complaints are the result of psychological turmoil, I try to identify the problem and defuse it before it intensifies into a real crises.

Even though teaching and counseling are central to basic nursing care, they are considered nonbillable skills. It is essential for nurses working in a nurse-managed clinic to provide these services. However, it becomes more costly to do so if a patient requires a half hour instead of 10 minutes. As an administrator, I must be concerned with productivity and fiscal management as well as patient care. I must encourage expeditious care that doesn't shortchange the patient. But because financial practicality is only a step away from the "busy doctor" trap, we walk a fine line between the two.

There are too few physicians working in small clinics and shelters. Moreover, it often is impractical to have specialists in these settings because it costs so much to maintain the technology they require. Consequently, nurse-managed clinics in poor urban and rural areas are an ideal way to increase access to health care for unserved and underserved populations.

Even so, I feel strongly that we must work hard to avoid the stereotype that nurse-managed care is fine for homeless people, but not for more affluent patients. I don't want the term *nurse-managed clinic* to become synonymous with second-class care. Ninety percent of primary care for any population can be delivered by nurses, and it's a perfectly viable alternative to traditional medicine. Still, specialized care has given us an entry and an opportunity to demonstrate our value. Already, there are nurse-managed clinics for women's health care and pain management. And nurse-managed centers are expanding their reach as nurse practitioners follow patients through hospitalization and even into the home. Such transitional care could become the unique territory of nurse-managed practices.

The delivery of basic primary care to all Americans is being given urgent priority. In this climate, nurse-managed health centers will evolve rapidly. At the same time, our challenge will be to remain sufficiently flexible to adapt to new demands.

My current role is almost entirely administrative. I make it a point to involve my staff in decisions on setting fees and in discussions about productivity and quality-of-care strategies. I encourage nurses who work here to give lectures, attend conferences, participate in research, and write articles. Above all, I don't want to promote the concept that they are the workers and I am the executive. That would be antithetical to the principles of a nurse-managed clinic.

In addition to my duties here, I'm on the advisory board of the Frontier Nursing Service, and I have two academic responsibilities. One of these is a joint appointment at the Columbia University School of Nursing, where I help develop nurse-managed centers and work in international nursing. I also have a joint appointment at the University of Utrecht in the Netherlands. There, as a visiting professor in nursing science, I'm helping develop master's and doctoral programs.

In nurse-managed clinics, nurse practitioners must be prepared to accept a large measure of independence. And they need enough confidence to make decisions. Both of these are acquired skills, and I recommend to my students that they begin developing them in an acute care setting and, perhaps, as a visiting nurse in home care. These experiences embrace a broad range of nursing care, sharpening the nurse's skills and making the autonomy of a nurse-managed clinic less threatening.

Nurse-managed clinics are ideal settings for increasing nursing career opportunities. Financially they represent important economies for the health care system. Yet, these clinics offer greater monetary rewards and enormous professional satisfaction to nurses. Those who choose this career path are in the unique position of being able to help create and shape an emerging field.

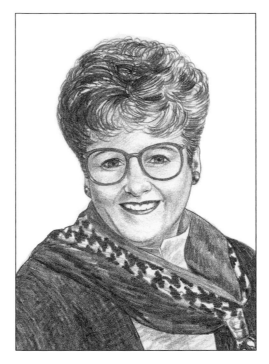

*Patricia Hinton Walker, PhD, MSN, RN, FAAN,
is associate dean, and director
of community-centered practice at the
University of Rochester School of Nursing,
Rochester, New York.*

Management and Administration

I worked in the office during the day, assisted in surgery in the evening, and often slept in the hospital at night. I was fresh out of college, and my introduction to nursing administration proved to be a trial by fire.

I hadn't bargained on administration; in fact, that first experience in my Kansas hometown was supposed to be nothing more than a summer job filling in for the vacationing director of nursing. But when she died rather suddenly after her return, I found myself moving into the position of an acting director and hospital administrator. For the next year or so, I was immersed in management and administration, and that abrupt change of plans set the stage for my whole career.

I'd gotten my BSN in 1966 from the University of Kansas, planning to become a cardiovascular clinical nurse specialist. However, that first job whetted my appetite for management—something I soon found I didn't know much about. Although my baccalaureate education included leadership courses, it contained little on real management. In self-defense, I began reading everything I could find on the subject, although most of it was related to business and not nursing.

That first job gave me a clinical background as well. In a small rural hospital, you treat whoever walks in the door: I've delivered babies, assisted in surgery and ER, and worked in geriatrics. All in all, that time in Kansas has helped me throughout my career, because I still do a lot of troubleshooting and consultation in rural settings. The chief advantage of beginning in such a small setting is that I had the authority—whether I felt ready for it or not—to change things. For instance, when I became acting director, I discovered that I had no people to work as aides in the community. My farm girl background told me to "grow my own," so I developed a course, taught it at night, and then hired my students. Less formally, I taught and believe I influenced the core of people who already were working for me.

During brief vacations, I escaped to Kansas City to be with my friends. They seemed lighthearted and playful, but I was dealing with life-and-death issues. I realized I was aging before my time. And despite all I was learning, I was certain that I didn't want to do my life's work in my hometown.

I changed direction and joined the Air Force as a cardiovascular nurse. The military exposed me to the larger clinical and cultural world, but its bureaucratic nature was frustrating. I saw so many things that needed changing, yet I felt powerless to do anything about them. I felt that in a different setting I could have influenced the process of change and outcomes.

After two years, I married and moved to Louisiana, where I took a job teaching psychiatric nursing in a diploma program. I also served on a committee to help prepare the school for accreditation. Before long, I went to work at the University of Arkansas at Fayetteville, where I helped develop a curriculum for a new associate degree program. Next we moved to Mississippi, and I found a part-time job as a staff nurse at a local hospital. The director of nursing asked me to help her develop infection-control and quality-assurance programs, then persuaded me to assume the duties of in-service director. In that capacity, I developed workshops for staff nurses, teaching management and supervisory skills, as well as conflict management. Soon I was conducting workshops at other facilities. Thus began my career in management consulting.

As a managerial and administrative consultant, I work with organizations that are under new management or need to change focus. My forte is helping the leaders develop a common vision of what they need to do. After helping identify problems, I assist the organization in developing solutions, or I may recommend other people who can help address the issues and problems.

Some people use the words *management* and *administration* interchangeably, but there are important distinctions between the two. Management encompasses planning and styles of exercising leadership. Conversely, administration involves structuring an environment and a process. Management involves proper allocation of resources, including people, capital, information, and equipment. Administration defines the systems — the policies and procedures — through which those resources are utilized.

While in Mississippi, I became involved at the state level with the American Nurses Association (ANA). In time, I was elected president of the Mississippi Nurses Association (MNA). This position called on all my leadership skills as I focused on using effective communication to create an impact on the political environment. I also worked to change our image from that of "nice nurses" to that of "smart businesswomen." Our mission didn't change, but our presentation and image did.

However, I soon discovered that managing a statewide volunteer organization is very different from management in a hospital. In the hospital, I was accustomed to having daily contact with people whose roles were more clearly delineated. But as president of MNA, I worked through a board of directors and learned to manage by motivating my volunteers, capitalizing on their interests and commitment to the profession.

I decided to work to work toward my master's degree at the University of Mississippi, focusing on medical-surgical nursing. Nursing administration wasn't available, and in any case, I felt that a solid clinical base would be more useful in my primary pursuits of teaching and administration. After completing my master's work, I went on for a doctorate in higher education and administration. Meanwhile, I worked as a director of nursing and assistant administrator at the Northwest Mississippi Regional Medical Center.

Next I was recruited to the deanship of the Mississippi College School of Nursing. The school formerly had difficulty in recruiting, retaining faculty, and maintaining its accreditation. It was definitely in need of new leadership and management.

As a dean, I learned about yet another aspect of management, which I put to further use when I was named associate dean of Emory University School of Nursing in Atlanta. This setting had BSN and MSN programs. A school can't be managed in the same way as a hospital. Most faculty members do not have a definitive job description, and they need a great deal of academic freedom — not the direction that many staff nurses require. Faculty members need support and guidance more than supervision. So, in an educational institution it's most important for the manager to create an environment in which these professional people can do the best possible job. I tried to anticipate the needs of my faculty, from computer support to secretarial staff, and I worked to establish a supportive climate that would facilitate student learning.

In my current position, which I've held since 1990, I have a dual title: associate dean and director of community-centered practice at the University of Rochester School of Nursing. As associate dean, I'm responsible with other deans for educational management of the school. Under my other title, I act as CEO of a professional corporation that develops entrepreneurial nursing practices in the community. For instance, we've developed a nurse-managed clinic and provide services in a group home for troubled adolescents. My two jobs overlap when it comes to developing faculty practice and establishing consultation teams to provide outreach services in rural areas.

Administrative opportunities for nurses can be found in hospitals, health departments, home health agencies, nursing corporations, educational institutions, and in occupational health. In a hospital, a nurse administrator would expect to start at the basic level of head nurse, supervising staff nurses, recommending policy and structural changes, and assisting in the implementation of changes. In a county health department, for another example, an entry-level administrator might work as a maternal-child health coordinator, arranging services that include immunizations and prenatal care.

The next administrative level is more complex, involving management responsibilities for entire services. Nurse administrators at this level might be clinical managers of a division, perhaps managing 25 nursing units with similar patients. They might manage in a county-wide or statewide organization, such as a visiting nurse association. While this work might involve management of a practice component, its scope is broad, emphasizing decision making and long-range planning responsibilities. At this level, day-to-day supervisory tasks are diminished.

Talented nurse administrators may advance to become hospital administrators, CEOs of nursing corporations, or deans and presidents of universities. Positions at this level will require strong decision-making abilities as well as the ability to achieve important goals through management.

I believe it's important for nurse administrators to begin in the trenches of their specialty: a hospital nurse administrator should start as a staff nurse; a dean should first be a faculty member and teach. Moreover, it's important to maintain that expertise and continue to build on it throughout a career, because more and more nurse administrators are retaining their clinical connections or perspective at the higher administrative levels.

I recommend that students who are interested in careers in administration get their BSNs and then look for entry-level leadership opportunities, such as might be available to a charge nurse. The next step up the academic ladder is to get an MSN, preferably in nursing administration. An option, for those who do not want to focus solely on administration, is to get a clinical master's degree as the main focus, as well as a functional emphasis in administration. Remember, however, that to move up to the top administrative levels, it's necessary to have substantial financial skills, which won't be adequately developed in a minor program. Yet another option that is becoming popular is to combine MN and MBA degrees.

Advanced education will pay off in the long run. While some nurses with specialized clinical practices may earn higher salaries than administrators, managers and administrators generally are paid more than the people who work for them. But of course, administrative jobs in the academic setting almost always pay less than equivalent jobs in a corporation or service setting.

The most successful administrators are energetic, visionary people who like to make things happen and who enjoy the challenge of improving things. They must be disciplined, with perseverance that will enable them to achieve long-range plans. These professionals also need enough self-confidence that they don't require constant praise or consistent feedback for a job well done. A bedside nurse enjoys the gratification of giving care and seeing a patient improve. Administrators seldom have such an opportunity for gratification.

Instead, they must be satisfied to see their work achieved — and recognized — through other people.

Good administrators can't be afraid to make decisions and, sometimes, mistakes. They can't be afraid to have people angry at them. Administrators often work in isolation and may not be able to discuss decisions with the people who work for them. In fact, I sometimes feel very alone in my work; sometimes I *am* very alone. I try to network with other professionals and seek other opinions, but I have to be prepared to live with my own decisions. I may suffer the pain of having to hurt or disappoint someone. Sometimes I am misunderstood because the need for confidentiality — and the threat of legal action — may prevent me from setting the record straight on facts that have been distorted.

Clearly, administrators can't be shrinking violets. But assertiveness and decision-making skills can be taught and practiced. It's more important to bring desire and willingness to a job, and then be prepared for the hard work to carry it through. I might keep nine-to-five office hours, but I carry my responsibilities 24 hours a day. On the other hand, I have an opportunity to watch people grow and to see my ideas become reality. I consider that a pretty fair trade.

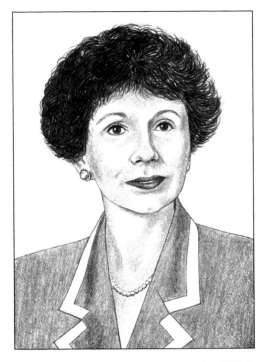

Madeline Zaworski, MBA, MSN, RN, CNAA,
is senior vice president
at Lorain Community Hospital,
Lorain, Ohio.

The Value of an MBA

When I entered nursing back in the 1960s, I saw it as one of few choices — along with teaching and becoming a nun — for a woman's career. At the time, I had little idea of how far I could go in my chosen career.

Fortunately, I soon found out — and I went on to advance my nursing education and to couple it with an MBA. That was an unusual path for a nurse, but it opened worlds of opportunities for me in nursing, health care management, and community involvement.

After graduating from a diploma program in 1968, I almost immediately set forth on my nontraditional nursing path. Within a year, at the ripe age of 21, I became the nurse manager of a coronary care unit. I worked under a physician who had been responsible for getting the unit up and running. He recognized my leadership abilities and facilitated an excellent first-line management learning experience for me. He proved to be a terrific role model and mentor.

The next year, I took another step upward when I participated as a nurse faculty member in a coronary care training program at Case Western Reserve University. There, I worked with an advanced practice nurse who recognized my teaching potential and encouraged me to obtain additional credentials.

I took her advice and returned to school in 1973. In 1976, I received a BSN from Kent State University. In 1979 I completed an MSN at Case Western, double-majoring in medical-surgical instruction and nursing administration. I worked in a variety of health care settings before returning in 1979 to Lorain Community Hospital. By then, I was 32 and ready for senior management.

Since then, I've worked as a nurse executive, although my titles have changed over the years. First I was nursing services administrator, then vice president of nursing, and two years ago was promoted to senior vice president — with no "of nursing" in the title.

I always have been considered a results-oriented leader and decision maker. I held a master's degree in nursing and felt confident in my abilities. But when I graduated from Case Western's Weatherhead School of Management in 1988 with an executive MBA, I discovered just what a business degree was worth. As a clinical expert and a knowledgeable businesswoman, I had more confidence in my abilities, and it was apparent that my colleagues had more respect for me. The combined result was that I had gained a distinct competitive advantage in my job. Even today, I am out of the ordinary in my job: I have an MBA and my title stops with the words "senior vice president." As vice president of nursing, I was responsible for only one major function. After I received my MBA, I became senior vice president, and other departments and additional corporate areas report to me as well.

My nursing training had prepared me with excellent interpersonal skills, as well as communication, prioritization, organization, and leadership skills. For me, enhancing these skills was the easy part of the MBA program. The harder part, because I had no undergraduate business degree, was learning advanced quantitative skills in business statistics, data processing, and finance. In the 1990s, those are skills a nurse executive needs.

Since the 1970s, it's been common for nurse executives to be included on the senior management teams of many hospitals, even though, especially in rural areas, those nurses might not even have BSNs. Is that acceptable? No, it is not acceptable in a health care environment in which we're dealing with reductions and a changing mix of RNs, LPNs, and aides. No, it is not acceptable when we're responsible for multimillion-dollar budgets. In this environment, nurse executives must justify budget variances, reduce overtime expenses, and perform complex cost-benefit analyses. These duties require business acumen that simply cannot be acquired in a diploma or AD program. It's possible to assign a business manager to work with the nurse manager, but it makes far more sense to bring the nurse manager up to business speed.

Such issues are indicative of the dramatic changes we are experiencing in health care. Costs have mushroomed in the wake of the technology boom that occurred during the last 15 years. When I started here in the late 1960s, the room rate was $39 a day. Now it's over $700 in the CCU. Health care is now an $800-billion industry that shouldn't be managed exclusively by business people and CEOs who don't understand the clinical side of health care delivery. If a nursing budget were left totally up to nonclinical executives, they would elect to eliminate RNs and rely on aides and other ancillary staff. Yet in the middle of all the current turmoil, our patients are getting sicker, and they require a level of care that a nursing aide is incapable of delivering or directing.

Nurse managers are in a tough position. The staff expects them to know the patients; the doctor expects them to make rounds; and the vice president expects them to manage a budget and participate in policy development. They need a business degree in order to make the transition from clinical practice to management.

For instance, a nurse manager orders a piece of equipment based on doctors' projected needs and meetings with salespeople. In taking this step, the nurse must understand the clinical reasons for the purchase and possess the business skills to negotiate intelligently. In addition, nurses are increasingly involved with case management. Under fixed-payment plans, they must work constantly with physicians to keep the costs of care within the reimbursement parameters. A business degree helps the nurse carry out those essential but basic financial aspects of the job.

An MBA carries clout, and I'm aware that my associates accord me a certain degree of respect because they know the training that lies behind those three letters. I can't fill in as an accountant, but because I understand financial theory and its application, I can talk the language. That's invaluable during budget negotiations, because it changes the ground rules and puts me in a much stronger bargaining position.

College curricula are changing in acknowledgement of the increased business skills needed by nurses in management and executive roles. It used to be that an MSN program in nursing administration incorporated a few classes in prioritization, budget preparation, organization, planning, and performance appraisal, but those courses were taught by members of the nursing faculty. Today, students take such classes as electives in the business school. And, within the last few years, combined-degree programs — either an MSN-MBA or an MSN-MPA — have been popping up all over the country. Although it takes a bit longer to get the combined degree, I recommend it for beginning nurse managers who aspire to senior vice presidencies or higher. The program provides advanced nursing courses and an understanding of nursing issues, as well as strong business preparation. Certainly a nurse *could* become a COO or CEO without an MBA, because experience and market demand are big factors. But the MBA is a powerful degree, and I don't think an MSN in nursing administration can supplant true business credentials.

The MBA has certainly helped me handle my current assignment, which is to lead the development of a corporate total quality management (TQM) program. The idea is that quality can be improved via process improvement by involving and empowering employees and by creating cross-departmental teamwork. As the responsible hospital executive, I assure that hundreds of employees are working in synchronization with the program, and I report on its progress to the board of directors.

My boss suggested I take this assignment since I believed in the concept and wanted an opportunity to put my MBA training to work with broader management responsibilities. And indeed, this project does combine the teamwork concepts I had acquired in nursing with the organizational behavior, strategic planning, statistics, and business-development theories I learned in the MBA program.

Another of my duties is overseeing our home health care department. For a health care financial management class I took as an MBA student, I wrote a proposal to start such a department, and I wound up implementing it at our institution. Organizationally, home health care personnel usually don't report to a nurse executive, but because my proposal and my business training were at work, I am responsible for this product line.

In another assignment, I worked with an outside consultant who reviewed our operating room. Now, I interface with the interdisciplinary committee that was formed to implement recommendations that have the potential for reducing the annual operating expense budget by several hundred thousand dollars.

I have drawn a conceptual framework, a series of concentric circles, that encompasses my different roles. Nursing is at the center. Immediately outside of that are hospital-wide responsibilities. Next are corporate activities. Then come community, regional, state, and national responsibilities. Some affiliations are nursing related, as with the executive committee of the Council on Nursing Administration of the American Nurses Association. Some are broader health care organizations such as the American College of Health Care Executives. Others encompass community functions. For instance, I currently chair the strategic planning committee of the Lorain County United Way and am a member of its board of trustees. Because that committee includes the president of the local community college and the board chair of a competing hospital, I feel this is a good example of how I've established myself and become recognized as a credible health care executive in this community.

For all that, I know biases still exist — some because I'm a woman, some because I'm a nurse. I remember one incident that occurred during a Chamber of Commerce meeting, when I was talking with a teacher who was acting superintendent of schools. He asked me about myself and my job, and concluded, "So you're a nurse. Why is a nurse doing chamber work?" I answered, "Well, you're a teacher. Why are you involved in chamber work?" Months later he apologized, but that is a perfect example of the stereotypes people immediately assign to nurses.

While I occasionally don my cap and uniform, I spend most of my time in a business suit. Instead of a stethoscope, I have a car phone, an executive secretary, and a briefcase. But I haven't lost my identity as a nurse, either. Now and then I make rounds, and if I am on a patient unit when the call bell rings, I answer it. I maintain these ties partly because I miss the clinical side of nursing, partly because I want to keep up with what's happening, and partly because my leadership style is to manage while walking around. Most important, I want to be a visible role model and mentor for my staff and encourage them to continue their education.

My schedule encompasses regular meetings with the hospital's board of trustees, the finance and personnel committees, and the medical staff. I'm active in various nursing organizations, both local and national. I often give guest lectures and currently precept two graduate students who are working on their MSNs. Last semester I had a student working on the combination MSN-MBA degree. In addition, I am an executive action team mentor for nonnursing MBA students.

Each week I meet with my directors — two directors of nursing and a director of home care — to tell them what's happening at the executive level, and I meet with all the leadership in my departments on a monthly basis. Twice a week I meet with the executive team, which consists of two vice presidents, two senior vice presidents, a COO, and a CEO. I'm the only woman member and the only executive with two master's degrees, both of which I consider necessary. The clinical master's (MSN) enables me to support proposals presented by MSN-prepared directors of nursing and clinical nurse specialists. The MBA is necessary for the credibility and skills factors already outlined in this chapter as preparation for a senior-level management/corporate position.

This job involves considerable long-range strategic planning. For instance, our institution is currently in consolidation negotiations with a local competing hospital, and I have a major role in preparing the what-if scenarios of such a consolidation. Part of my job has to do with strictly senior management issues: approval of capital purchases over $10,000; developing the hospital's strategic plan; and final approval for the hospital budget. Because I am the only woman on our executive team, I work particularly hard to be a role model and mentor for women managers and medical staff members. I regret that I didn't know enough about alternatives early in my career, so I spend time encouraging young women to pursue advanced degrees and to see beyond their current circumstances.

Looking forward is necessary for me, even at an advanced level. I think the typical hierarchy of department managers seen in hospitals today will be reconfigured as health care providers become more cross-functional. In that scenario, the position of vice president of nursing might not require a nursing degree, and it might not even exist as the job is defined today. Therefore, I want to broaden my experience base to include other assignments and departments. I believe that a good leader with team-building skills can manage in a variety of settings. I maintain a nursing image because nursing plays an integral role in a health care institution. Indeed, combined skills in nursing and business place me in a prime position to become a CEO. At this point in my career that's a goal I believe is attainable because of the opportunities that will result from health care reform. Providing quality care in the face of cost containment can be done quite easily with intimate knowledge of these two disciplines.